Healing through
Cranial Osteopathy

Healing through
Cranial Osteopathy

Tajinder K. Deoora

FRANCES LINCOLN

Frances Lincoln Limited

4 Torriano Mews

Torriano Avenue

London NW5 2RZ

www.franceslincoln.com

British Library Cataloguing in Publication Data

A catalogue record for this book is available from the British Library

ISBN 0 7112 1781 5

Set in Fairfield LH Light

Printed and bound in Singapore

1 2 3 4 5 6 7 8 9

Foreword

First let me say: this book is very honest, complete and a joy to explore. Tajinder Deoora has taken on a challenge that most osteopaths would find impossible. How does one explain osteopathy to people outside the profession? In this book Tajinder has used all her gifts of communication, language and experience to weave the principles and the practice of osteopathy into an understandable format. The reader can sit back and take a journey through the 'inside' of osteopathy.

The principles of healing that lie behind osteopathy are very different from those of other schools of medicine and healing. Perhaps osteopathy's greatest gift is a dedication to uncovering new horizons in the natural laws of healing. This text is really a first of its kind: it will open new horizons for the reader and shed light upon the daily practice of osteopathy.

James Jealous, D.O.

Author's note

Osteopathy to me is a very sacred science. It is sacred because it is a healing power through all nature.

Dr Andrew Taylor Still

Throughout my years as a cranial osteopath, patients have continually asked me for explanations of what I was doing. Since it was difficult to talk and treat at the same time, I looked for something they could refer to. I discovered there was nothing that was appropriate, and I eventually realized that I was going to have to write this book.

Throughout the book I have tried to describe the concepts of osteopathy and primary respiration, as I understand them, through clinical settings. In the text the osteopath is referred to as 'she', since I am a woman, and, to avoid confusion, the patient, unless named, is referred to as 'he'. Although the patients' names have been altered, the cases described are real and typical of those seen in my clinic.

Many people have helped me in the writing of this book. First and foremost I would like to thank my very dear friend Dr Christine Page for her constant support and invaluable advice and direction.

My sincere thanks go to all my colleagues who very kindly shared their ideas and comments on each chapter. In particular, I would like to thank Peter Armitage for his contribution in the early chapters and his paper on 'Tensegrity', Susie Booth and Tim Williams for their reviews of the text, Christian Sullivan for pointing me in the right direction when needed, and Dr James Jealous for sharing his insights.

My heartfelt thanks go to Stuart Korth, my dear colleague who inspired me to study primary respiration in the first place, and continues to guide me even now.

My thanks also go to my friend and constant support Jeetej Singh for lifting my spirits and helping with my time schedules.

I would also like to thank Judith Warren, my editor, for her guidance. She has been absolutely wonderful to work with.

My warm appreciation goes to Chris Ronaldson, Valerie Greenwood and Johnny Rothman, and to all my friends and patients who contributed in their own way.

Finally, I would like to give my deepest thanks and gratitude to my loving parents and family, for their patience, nurturing and constant support.

Introduction

The doctor of the future will give no medicine, but interest his patient in the care of the human frame, in diet, and in the cause and prevention of disease.

Thomas Edison

Max's beginning

Julie was on the verge of tears. With dark rings under her eyes, she looked haggard and was utterly exhausted. Julie was a new mother and did not know what to do with her fractious son. She had tried feeding him, rocking him, taking him for a drive, rubbing his tummy, giving him gripe water, a dummy, changing his nappy, but nothing seemed to work for more than a few minutes. She was now desperate. The six-week-old baby would not be consoled and yelled constantly. It was obvious that neither mother nor child had slept for any decent period since the birth.

Julie had been waiting patiently and quietly as we ran late. It was Friday. That meant a very busy afternoon in the children's clinic at the British School of Osteopathy in London. I had recently entered the third year and was only just beginning to cope with normal clinic days when we saw adults. Children, on the other hand, I had reservations about. They were a force to be reckoned with. For a start they did not speak, they looked at you with unnerving directness and they were not as obliging as adults when you wanted to examine them. With my inexperience and lack of confidence in handling babies, I had deliberately avoided Julie with her irritable infant. But Stuart Korth, who ran the children's clinic, had other ideas for me!

So I took Julie and her tiresome infant to the consulting room. listening to her story, I did not know who I felt more sorry for: the desperate mother who felt powerless to help her baby, or the poor baby, whose only means of expression was to scream, kick and lie exhausted, recouping his energies before the whole process began again.

I tried to find out what the matter was, but each time I tried examining Max, I was thwarted. He would not let me undress him. He would not let me anywhere near his head, and he kicked his legs too strongly for me to find any other area of contact. Max was only interested in screaming his head off. Fortunately, help and teaching were at hand. Stuart instructed the mother to encourage the baby to feed at the breast, whilst cradling him. I was instructed to place one hand on the stomach and the other under

Max's bottom so that it was on top of a number of layers of winter clothing and thick nappy. Then Stuart placed his hands on top of mine, and we waited. After a while (when I was not able to feel very much, with Stuart doing all the work) a total transformation occurred. The baby was no longer fractious. In fact, he had fallen asleep. His breathing changed – it became deeper and seemed to be happening throughout the body rather than just at the chest. The redness from the face had gone, replaced by a much healthier glow.

And there he lay for quite some time. Both the mother and I were intrigued. What had happened to bring about this transformation? How was it possible for it to take place on so many levels – for Stuart to have felt anything through my hand and so many layers of clothing and nappy, let alone carry out a treatment? How could he have brought about this change, only from putting a hand on Max's bottom?

My journey learning about health through 'cranial osteopathy' had begun.

Margaret's last months

I began to work with Margaret just after graduating. I was qualified with all the right theories and techniques at my disposal. Very quickly I realized that now my real teachers would be the patients.

Margaret had developed cancer shortly after her husband died, about three years before she came to see me. She was 67 years old and had done well with her life, maintaining her positive attitude. Unfortunately, she was now beginning to feel rather frail, weak and tired. She ached everywhere and her specialist was giving her morphine to allay the pain. This helped, but not enough. Her GP advised Margaret to have some cranial treatment, in an effort to make her feel more comfortable. She had been attending every week for the last nine months and although the cancer did not change, she felt more at ease. With each treatment aimed at supporting her inner health and vitality and subtly easing the areas of immobility, Margaret felt better. She did not suffer the intensity of pain quite so much, and generally felt more able to cope. She knew that she was dying as the cancer continued to take hold, but now what mattered most to her was the quality of her rather restricted everyday life, and the gentle methods of osteopathy helped. Somehow, the body was induced to release the right chemicals for easing the pain and releasing stress patterns of the body. In the last month Margaret was unable to get to the practice and we took turns to visit her at home, where she died peacefully.

Both Max and Margaret had benefited from osteopathy, but for different reasons: Max was helped to start his new life through attaining comfort within his body and Margaret gained some relief and restfulness in her final months. Osteopathy had in both cases enabled the body to be at ease, and to find in osteopathic terms a greater degree of 'health'. For Max, this meant helping his body to cope with the trauma of birth. For Margaret, this meant that she was eventually able to leave her cancer-ridden body at peace with herself.

Why see an osteopath?

Most people seek help from an osteopath to deal with pain, but there are other reasons too. Feelings of tiredness, headaches, bloated stomach, period problems or tension in the neck are just some symptoms which reveal a deviation from the usual state of wellbeing. People generally seek help when they 'don't feel right' or have been given a diagnosis of a condition, with the assumption that they have to 'live with it'.

The concepts of osteopathy and cranial osteopathy were the products of the lifetime's work of two men. Dr Andrew Taylor Still gave us osteopathy, whilst Dr William Garner Sutherland's gift was the discovery of the 'Breath of Life' and the role this played in healing through osteopathy in the cranial field. Parts of the osteopathic journey of these great men are described in appendix 2

Dr Andrew Taylor Still's osteopathy

Dr Andrew Taylor Still (1828–1917) discovered the art and science of osteopathy and founded its first school at Kirksville, Missouri in 1892. He was a frontier doctor who, having lost three children to meningitis, searched for a better system of healing than was available. A great humanitarian and medical pioneer, Dr Still had a remarkable understanding of the workings of the human body. His ideas and practice were so radical and imaginative that it is difficult to place them in the medical context of the period. In fact, his ingenious insights that the body contains its own drugstore releasing chemicals and transmitters in response to injury and disease have been subsequently vindicated.

The philosophy of osteopathy, as expressed by Still, was extensive, taking into account the structure of the human body as well as the universal forces presiding over nature. These forces were interconnected and their expression of life was through mind, matter and motion that had order and intention. Still emphasized the body's capacity for movement and his conviction that the body's healing capacity can be facilitated by working on the inter-relationships between its structure, function and motion form the basis of osteopathy. Still's crucial idea that motion plays a primary role in health and disease was, and remains, grossly underestimated.

Still called the discipline osteopathy 'because you begin with the bones' – *osteo* is Latin for bone. He was emphatic that disease was an effect of a disturbance in the natural flow of blood. Nerves were seen to play a large part in contributing to this since their excitation causes the muscles to contract and therefore compress the veins returning blood to the heart. The bones, then, were the starting point, to be used as levers to relieve pressure on the blood vessels and nerves.

The Breath of Life

One of Still's students at Kirksville in the 1900s was Dr William Garner Sutherland, who pioneered 'cranial osteopathy' or osteopathy in the cranial field.

This came about when he saw a skull, or cranium, whose 26-odd bones had been separated. He noticed that the surfaces of two of these joined in such a way that they resembled the gills of a fish. Sutherland speculated that, like the gills, the cranial bones were designed for a breathing motion. Contrary to the view then held, that the bones of the skull were fused and immovable in adulthood, he realized there was movement between the joints or sutures. To Sutherland, this implied a form of respiratory mechanism of the structures contained within the cranium. When the osteopath places her hands on either side of the head, it feels as if it is expanding and contracting in response to this repiratory mechanism.

Sutherland's greatest contribution to osteopathy was his insight into the force that manifested life: this he called the 'Breath of Life'. Other traditions have their own terms for this life force: the Chinese, for example, refer to it as 'Qi', the Indians name it 'Prana', while homeopaths call it 'Vital Force'.

He saw the Breath of Life as the original animating essence of all the inherent motions of the body. What originally started off as a diligent study into the rhythmic 'breathing' movements of cranial bones led to the discovery of a whole series of rhythmic tissue and fluid motions. Among these he found the fluctuating motion of the cerebrospinal fluid (CSF) of the brain and spinal cord, while the brain itself also demonstrated rhythmic micro-motions. He also found that the sacrum (the large bone at the end of the spine) moved independently from its two neighbouring pelvic bones. In addition, special membranes called meninges linked the head and pelvis, and therefore motion or tension could also be carried within these. The culmination of all the movements of the various tissues and structures corresponded to those felt at the cranial bones and all occurred simultaneously. These he named 'primary respiration'.

The rhythmic, tidal motions instigated by the Breath of Life were felt throughout the body and Sutherland regarded them as essential to life and physiology. As every function of the body has a control centre in the brain, it was primary respiration that seemed to influence all the other physiological processes of life, including that which we know as breathing. And so, the motions of primary respiration were seen to provide access to the essential processes that heal and regulate the body.

Sutherland, in his search for the origins of the phenomenon of primary respiration, saw a profound principle of life at work – that life is manifested in motion. Since muscles were not involved in moving the cranial bones, these and the motions of the brain and cerebrospinal fluid were the physical manifestations of the life force itself. The Breath of Life was responsible for setting into motion the natural rhythms of the different structures of the body. It was seen as the universal intention in action, which provided the organizing principles of the universe and also the interconnectedness of the physical body and the environment.

The potency of the Breath of Life

During the process of development in embryology, the Breath of Life provided the 'initiative spark' or ignition for the engine of life. It was seen to generate function within the form that it had created, and was the organizer for the central nervous system and its fluid. As the body developed its bioelectric, biomolecular and biomechanical nature, the Breath of Life instigated the different rhythms of these components. And, at the time of birth, the impetus to breathe air and the individualization of the body occurred with further ignition from the Breath of Life, thus setting the newborn on its journey. Sutherland saw the Breath of Life being received by the cerebrospinal fluid and it carried with it a subtle but very powerful force or 'potency'. This was the driver for the rhythms generated by the Breath of Life and could be felt by skilled hands.

This idea of the potency of the Breath of Life is a fundamental principle in the cranial concept and it is an effective tool in many therapeutic procedures used by osteopaths in the cranial field. This is related to the interconnecting nature of the Breath of Life, and its generation of the rhythms that are expressed by every single cell in the body (see figure 1). The rhythmic motions under the influence of the potency of the Breath of Life are used by osteopaths to encourage an interchange between the circulatory systems of various nourishing substances required for the sustenance and regeneration of the cells. This interchange is possible because the brain and spinal cord containing the cerebrospinal fluid are in close proximity to the membranes of blood vessels as well as to the lymphatic channels.

Sutherland emphasized that the cranial concept was osteopathy and therefore a science. 'It is not an integral part of osteopathy, it is osteopathy. It is not a "therapy" . . . for this is a science that deals with the natural forces.' The study of natural forces provides the foundation for some of the basic principles of osteopathy, which the osteopath will aim to effect when she facilitates the natural healing processes.

Basic principles in osteopathy

Osteopathy is a system of medicine that is based on the science of living anatomy and physiology, both in the normal and abnormal states. It is a 'natural' medicine in the sense that it relies entirely on the natural laws that govern the function of the body, as outlined below.

• **The body interacts constantly with its surroundings** and therefore needs to live in favourable conditions, where pollution and harmful substances do not saturate the atmosphere. We rely on our environment for air, food and water. Nutrition adequate in fluids, vitamins, minerals, proteins, fats and carbohydrates is vital for the physiological processes of the body. Advanced technology and today's fast lifestyle seem increasingly to compromise these essential aspects of our survival.

- **The body has the ability to maintain a constant internal environment so that the vital processes of life can be sustained.** Through the process known as 'homeostasis' the organs and tissues of the body play their part in various self-regulating mechanisms.
- **The body has the ability to protect itself in the face of offending organisms and poisons.** It is capable of making its own remedies against disease and other toxic conditions. The immune system plays a large part in these self-healing mechanisms.

These ideas are common to all systems of medicine. However, where osteopathy differs is in emphasizing how important it is for the body to be physically balanced in order to function at its best.

Osteopathy considers the importance of structural and functional inter-relationships of the body to be vital to the maintenance of health and wellbeing. While recognizing the effects of disease on the body, osteopaths believe that faulty functioning of the body structures can increase susceptibility to ill health. This also works the other way: if you are already suffering from ill health, then recovery can be maximized by normalizing the body structure and function. In relation to this, the following factors are essential for healthy function:

- **Movement of the body fluids is essential for transport of substances.** An unhindered supply of blood will ensure the transport of oxygen and other nutritive substances to the area that requires them. Equally, the venous and lymphatic circulations will ensure that waste products of the tissues are carried away for their elimination.
- **Nerves play a crucial part in controlling blood supply.** Nerves control the diameter of the muscles of the blood vessel walls. As a result, blood flow to the organs and other structures can be altered by the extent of nerve stimulus. Therefore blood flow through a constricted vessel will, over a period of time, affect the function of that structure.
- **Nerves control the activities of the body.** Certain parts of the body not only manifest disease but can also contribute to it through nerve circuits.

Nerves send and receive signals via pathways from the spinal cord within the vertebral column and the body parts in two ways:

- Through the spinal nerves, which control the activity of the muscles and joints of the body.

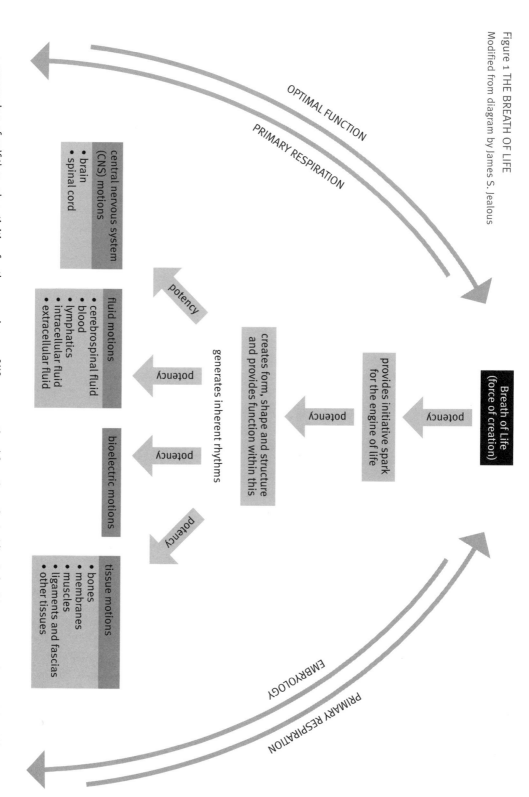

Figure 1 THE BREATH OF LIFE
Modified from diagram by James S. Jealous

14

• Through the autonomic spinal pathways that interact with the organs and other internal structures; these pathways are known as 'reflexes'.

Thus, a problem in an organ (viscera) may be identified in its reflex component at the spine or other body part (soma). A diseased gall bladder, for instance, may reflect as pain in the right shoulder, through the viscero-somatic reflex. Equally, a problematic area in the spine may affect the function of its related internal organ through the somato-visceral reflex.

• **Ill health occurs when the normal ability of the body to adapt to a situation is disrupted, or when environmental factors overwhelm its defence systems.** In looking for the cause of discomfort, osteopathy recognizes the importance of 'cause and effect' relationships, over a period of time. For example, an old football injury (the cause) might have strained the ligaments of the knee, thus destabilizing it (the effect). Over time, the altered weight-bearing through this joint (adaptation) has a knock-on effect on the way the back behaves during activities such as walking. So the recent low back pain (the most recent effect) is indirectly related to the old football injury.

Motion, structure and function in the living body

As we have seen, osteopathy emphasizes the importance of the structure, motion and function of the body in relation to health and disease. It is therefore important to appreciate the way in which osteopaths understand and work with the body's capacity for movement, as this is crucial to diagnostic and therapeutic procedures.

Osteopathy is a science that is based on the study of structure and function as it is in the living body. 'Living' is the key word here; the principal feature of a living body is that it is dynamic and in perpetual motion. Compare the wood in your table with the wood in the tree outside as it dances with the breeze. The table wood is inert, but the living tree has movement within its structures. All living things express their function through motion within their tissues. Therefore the study of living anatomy and physiology is the study of the relationship between structure, function and motion. Osteopaths love motion – it is the key to their work.

Through her specialized sense of touch, the osteopath feels for motion within the tissues of the body. She will perceive an altered degree or quality of motion as an altered physiology within that structure. This indicates that part of the body has an imbalance in function which, since all body parts are interdependent, will affect its total function. So interpreting the body's motion in its range, quality and pattern is of prime importance to the osteopath.

Movement and motion

The body is designed to move and it does this on many levels. We live our lives through the body's ability to perform activities consciously and yet maintain its life processes without us being aware of them. The different types of tissues within the body have different types of movement and they perform their functions in two ways:

- Through movements we can and do initiate, and are able to stop at will. We can move either the whole body or certain parts in order to perform various activities. These are 'voluntary' movements that occur through the action of muscles on the joints.
- Through movements within the body that we do not initiate, and which we cannot stop, but which are continual. These are known as 'inherent motions' because they are automatic and innate. They are the motions of the cells of the body and the fluid present within and around them. Because of the fluid and membranous nature of the body, these motions can be felt throughout the body by trained hands.

All types of movements and inherent motions of the body influence each other.

The motions of primary respiration

The inherent motions of primary respiration are modified by genetic, nutritional and environmental factors as well as:

- Birth strain
- Illness and disease
- Problems of the muscles and joints
- Posture
- Emotions
- Accidents and trauma, especially at the head and pelvis
- Stress

In chapter two I will look in more detail at the physiological structures and features of the inherent motions and primary respiration, and how this affects the body.

Osteopathy using primary respiration is a precise science that bridges physical medicine and mind-body medicine. This is because the body reflects its owner's life; it shows the effects of physical activity, illness, infection and emotional traits. Through assessing the active movements, inherent motions and hence the structure and function of the body, the osteopath can address many of the stress and strain patterns listed above and so facilitate the well-being of her patient.

The healing power of nature

Being well means that the body can respond appropriately and efficiently to any situation that disturbs the normal state of affairs, without us being distressed by it. Mechanisms such as the regulation of body temperature in the face of changing weather, normalizing of blood sugar levels or blood pressure are automatic. The functions of the body may be regarded as a series of integrated but interdependent biochemical processes that are self-regulating. These myriad processes, however, do not work in isolation and are considered to be under the guidance of an innate Intelligence. Although osteopathy is a science based on the understanding of anatomy, physiology and the biochemical and pathological processes of health and disease, osteopaths acknowledge that the 'life force' is the driver of all life processes and is ever-present.

The same Breath of Life that created our form and function is the director of the healing processes of the body. In response to illness or trauma, it brings about the mechanisms of adaptation, so that we, as a whole, are not destroyed. When the body is exposed to substances that harm it, the healing processes behave in a perfectly ordered manner. Think of what happens when you cut your finger. The injured area swells up and the increased flow of blood brings with it factors that provide nutrition and fight infection. The formation of scar tissue walls off the area, thereby delaying the spread of bacteria and the toxic products of injury to the rest of the body. Similarly, when we have an accident, the body changes the energy of trauma into something that it can deal with; an effect may be a broken bone, for example. Equally, when we are emotionally upset, the body 'heals with time'. These processes of involuntary readjustment, of self-regulation and self-healing, are well organized and constitute the healing power of nature and we take them for granted. Nothing man-made can compare to these – the broken bone will heal, but if a china plate is broken, it will never mend again. The healing power of nature is an extremely powerful force.

What is 'health'?

It is interesting to note that there is no real definition for health. Most medical authorities define health as an absence of disease rather than a presence of something that is given. Dorland's medical dictionary defines health as 'A state of optimal physical, mental and social wellbeing, and not merely the absence of disease and infirmity.' What do these aspects of 'wellbeing' consist of?

The physical plane relates to the physiological, biochemical and biomechanical structure of the body. The mental aspect relates to the psychological and emotional mind state, whilst the social wellbeing may relate to the collective, communal level as well as the spiritual or subconscious levels, although all aspects are inter-related.

For an osteopath, health is an optimal state of structural integration and cohesion of the physical body, mind and spirit. However, apart from being a self-contained unit that has the ability for homeostasis and self-healing, the body also interchanges with the immediate external environment. Becker describes this symbiotic relationship as the 'bioenergy field of health'. Because each person is different, health will be unique to each individual and will vary with age and changing circumstances. Health in a toddler is different from when he reaches puberty or turns sixty, just as it varies after he has recovered from pneumonia. Osteopaths who use primary respiration detect health in the patient as 'a palpable sensation of a quiet, rhythmic feeling of total interchange between the patient's body and his biosphere, without any areas of restriction, impaction, trauma or stress', as Becker writes in his book *Life in Motion*. These dynamic, alternating, rhythmic motions of primary respiration remain throughout life and for the osteopath they are the expression of the ever-present inner health of the patient.

How does the body come to be unwell?

Wellness is dependent not only on our genetic constitution but also to a large extent on how we take care of ourselves. However, most of us live lifestyles where demands for performance are high – speed and efficiency dominate. In order to maintain this we turn to habits that do not nurture us. Excess of alcohol, stimulants such as tea, coffee or nicotine, mixed with little sleep, lack of fun and relaxation plus neglect of spiritual needs, will if continued long enough make us unwell. The body warns us through symptoms such as headaches or disturbed bowel motions. But, most of us ignore these signs and so tend to function from a state of sub-health. Not ill enough to take a day off work, and yet not well enough to work or play to our full potential. This is also because the body has continually adapted to the effects of different stressful situations throughout life. Known as 'stressors', these may be infections, physical or emotional trauma, postural habits or any other taxing problems. When successive stressors exceed the body's ability to recover from them, it moans with discomfort, tension or fatigue amongst other symptoms.

An osteopath would regard a sinus infection or a strained back from bending awkwardly as effects of other underlying causes. Factors such as birth strain, previous illnesses or injuries cause the whole body to respond with complex and far-reaching effects on the specific and the general state of health. She will look at the mechanisms leading to the current dysfunctional state. It does not matter if the ailment is one of pain, infection or a general sense of being unwell – the important thing is how did this state come to be? So the osteopath will investigate both the immediate cause and the various factors that predisposed the body to be vulnerable to that condition.

Infections

An infection is usually regarded as the invasion of the body by bacteria, fungi or viruses. We are, however, surrounded by bugs all the time, so why is it that some people are susceptible whilst others are not? Indeed, the body is always full of bugs yet these do not create a perpetual infection. We seem only to succumb to them at certain times. Quite often we get non-specific symptoms, which are frequently labelled as 'viral' infections and yet the blood tests are clear.

We generally tend to become vulnerable to infection and disease when our immunity is reduced. This causes cellular changes so that the body's defences cannot adequately deal with a bug. Our inner balance is affected by any number of things, including accidents, distress, lack of love, nourishment, rest and relaxation. When combined with the ecological effects of polluted air, impure water, use of chemicals and preservatives in food, the toxicity overburdens the resources of the body. Eventually, this depletes the immune system and the body becomes inefficient at dispensing with infectious agents.

Pain

Pain in the body is the effect, rather than the cause, of some underlying process. It generally relates to an alteration in the mechanics of the body structure. When not related to a disease process, it is often due to inflammation and may be associated with some dysfunction of the joints or severe contraction of a muscle. Unless related to immediate trauma, it is very rare that a pain arises in the joints or muscles on a one-off basis; there is usually a precipitating factor that finally limits the body's ability to recover. Back pain in pregnancy, for example, may well be from an unresolved strain in the pelvis as a result of an old fall.

In children, a lot of problems can be traced back to unresolved birth strains. Because the cranial bones are so malleable they can easily overlap during the birth process. In most cases this is of no consequence. Sometimes, however, a complicated labour can bring about general compression in the body, especially of the bones at the base of the skull. This can leave the whole body system so irritable that the baby may become inconsolable. Max, whom we met at the beginning of this chapter, was just such a baby.

The right choice for you?

Osteopaths recognize and use normal medical procedures such as X-rays, MRI scans, laboratory investigations and so on and are respectful of the need for surgical interventions when necessary. They do, however, make their own diagnosis. Although osteopaths do not rely on medications, drugs, pressure or reflex points, they can work alongside any therapeutic system that employs such approaches.

What distinguishes osteopathy from other forms of physical medicine is the attention given to tracing the source of the problem, whilst taking into consideration the effects of the patient's previous history on the health of tissues. The diagnostic and therapeutic procedures place emphasis on restoring motion, in the broadest sense, within the body. Accordingly, the treatment is based on giving support while discomfort persists, and on strengthening affected areas so as to improve the body's overall function. Restoring motion assists this, which in turn helps the body's capacity to heal itself.

The beauty of osteopathy is that it is so individual. Since the human body is a dynamic force that is never static, no two treatments are ever the same – each treatment is tailor-made. Most people associate osteopathic treatment with 'clicks' and 'cracks' coming from parts of the body they never knew existed or indeed were capable of making such a noise! In healing through osteopathy in the cranial field, the osteopath reads and seeks to influence the physiological rhythmic motions discovered by Sutherland, which will, in turn, affect the body's overall functioning. It is a deceptively gentle but profound means of body treatment, involving a light, refined touch which acts on the subtle stresses and strains throughout the body.

Osteopathy can be practised in many different ways according to the choice of both the practitioner and the patient. The use of primary respiration is particularly useful where the person needs very gentle procedures with minimal handling, as we saw with Margaret, the lady with cancer, at the beginning of the chapter. This means that even very sick people can benefit, especially as the treatment rarely contradicts any other form of medicine they might be receiving. In fact, today many osteopaths work alongside orthodox medicine and many general practitioners refer their patients for osteopathy. Because it is such a gentle and non-intrusive method of working with the body, treatment can be given at any age. Osteopathy is effective in its own right at treating specific conditions related to trauma or disease, and as preventive medicine for maintaining a person's wellbeing and good health.

Why see an osteopath who works with primary respiration?

The Breath of Life is the very essence which allows us to live to our fullest potential:

• To engage with life fully
• To enjoy life fully
• To express ourselves fully

When the rhythms of primary respiration are not being expressed fully by the body, we feel disharmony, distress and disease. The way we live our life often causes us to take up inappropriate postures or insufficient time to rest and recover from an exhausting work period, accident or emotional trauma. These influence the motions of primary respiration so that the natural healing processes cannot function to their fullest extent. The osteopath's job is to clear any restrictions or blocks within all the compartments of the body and she engages the potency of the Breath of Life to enable her to achieve this. She can perceive the Breath of Life entering into the body from the outside and giving potency to the different rhythms of the different tissues. This, in turn, facilitates a harmonious interchange of nutritious substances and a balance of both structure and function, so facilitating the full potential for health.

Chapter one

The structure and function of the body

The miracle of life expresses itself in motion and movement. Life in the body is working as a unified whole mechanism to manifest health, to resist and combat disease, and to correct or adapt to trauma. I, as a physician, and my patient, as an individual, are endowed with life, which manifests itself as motion and movement. As physicians, it is self-evident that we can use this manifested motion and movement as keys to diagnosis and treatment in the care of our patients.

Rollin E. Becker, D.O.

We experience life through the different functions and activities of the body. We work, play sports, cry, give birth, think, are touched or moved by certain things. We garden, read, philosophize, sing, eat or meditate. When this ultimate instrument is fine-tuned, there is cohesion within the self and the world around, so that we experience the symphony of life to its fullest. When filled with vitality, energy and movement we feel connected with the world and 'in tune'.

We can work to our optimum only when the body's structural and functional inter-relationships are in balance. Osteopathy considers these to be inseparable in health and disease. Just as the structure of the body will affect its function, so too will the function affect its structure. The influence of structure on function is easy to see: for example, in a sprained ankle joint that makes walking difficult. The effect of function on the structure is more difficult to envisage, but comes to light when we see how the body has to adapt to the effects of a disease or injury. For example, as a result of a car accident, you may have a whiplash injury where the joints of the neck become unstable, thereby trapping a nerve. Because it cannot function adequately, after a period of time the muscles supplied by the nerve become wasted, so altering their structure. In this manner, the structure of the body and its function cannot be separated.

The structural coherence of the body

The structure of the body is a marvellous piece of engineering that has enabled us to evolve from being on all fours to an upright position. This evolutionary process is mirrored in every individual's growth and development.

When we visualize the structure of the body, we automatically think in terms of the bony skeleton that is 'held together' by muscles and ligaments. However, the structure is made up of many different tissues, which form its various parts but function with the integrity and coherence of a complete unit. The various tissues that make up the body are:

• Hard tissues such as bone and cartilage
• Soft tissues such as skin, muscles, ligaments, fascias, tendons, membranes
• Fluids such as the cellular fluids, blood, lymph and the cerebrospinal fluid (CSF)

The structure of the framework is formed by the skeleton, which is often thought of as the body's architectural foundation. It is built through the attachments of ligaments, muscles and the complex interconnecting matrix of fascias and membranes. Fascia is a special membrane of fibro-elastic tissue that knits the body together. It lies under the skin in very thin bands or sheets and interconnects the whole body by forming various pockets and folds to envelop muscles, tendons, joints, nerves, blood and lymph channels, the organs and all internal structures. This framework provides support, stability, strength and form to the body, whilst enabling us to adapt to our external environment.

Our survival as a species has depended on our ability to remain upright. In so doing, the compression forces of gravity are brought to bear on the body. Whilst we were in the uterus this was not important, as we were surrounded by fluid. And it is interesting to note that our bony skeleton only develops after the nerve and blood pathways have been established. Then, after the birth, the muscles will grow with the skeleton so that as the baby learns to crawl and walk the bones and muscles get stronger. In this way, the skeleton responds to the demands of gravity, weight bearing and movement – all forces having compressive effects on the body.

The structural integrity of the body is maintained by its soft tissues, which 'hold it together'. This can be likened to strips of wood tied with a rope, to make a raft floating on the water. If the rope is too loose then the raft is unstable and the wood spreads. If it is too tight, it causes the bits of wood to buckle. The tension needs to be just adequate to hold the raft together, in the face of the flow of water. The soft tissues similarly keep us upright in the face of gravity by maintaining a degree of tension or tone.

In his paper on 'Tensegrity: the role of tensional force in human structure', Peter Armitage writes, 'This vision of the soft tissues of the body as an all-embracing tension network, constantly charged [and] self-adjusting, permits a different view of other body phenomena . . . there is a structural homeostasis, as much as a physiological homeostasis, that is being constantly maintained . . . the body is in a state of constantly changing equilibrium, so its physical and

23

chemical processes are perpetually adapting and readjusting. It maintains harmony by working in counterpart mechanisms that respond to the fluctuating environment produced by cells, tissues and outside forces. The mechanisms of homeostasis allow us to get hot and cool down, for example, whilst forces in the body pull and push.' The latter principle can be seen when the arm is bent, so that the muscles at the front contract and tighten, whilst those at the back relax and lengthen. Similarly, Armitage explains that the body must maintain harmony with the external environment, and here tension becomes the dynamic counterpart to the compressive forces of life (gravity and weight bearing). The forces of tension and compression always coexist in the body.

The body adapts to the environmental compression forces through the constant interplay in tension within its network of soft tissues. The membranes, muscles, ligaments and fascias all blend and interweave in various directions to form a vast and complex 'tensional network'. The beauty of this mechanism is that any weight on the body can be dispersed uniformly. An example of this can be seen in the spine, which is normally regarded as a column of square bones with the discs between them acting as shock absorbers. However, the strength and elasticity of the ligaments, and the extensive length and breadth of the fascias with their different planes ensures that the vertebral column does not bear weight like a stack of blocks. The compressive forces on the spine are evenly distributed thanks to the constant setting and adjustment of tension in the membranous network. This network continues at deeper levels within the body through the cranial and spinal membranes, which connect the spine to the skull and pelvis. It is through these membranes that the osteopath can feel the tensional support of the sacrum and follow it right up to the cranium.

Tension is maintained throughout the body due to its fluid nature; fluid pervades all kinds of tissues, be they brain, muscles, membranes – even bone contains fluid. The boundary of a fluid-filled cell is its membranous wall. It maintains its shape due to the fluid pushing outwards against this wall. Numerous cells together form a tissue and this becomes specialized to form an organ, such as the heart. The organ is then enclosed by a membranous capsule and sits within the fluid compartment of the body. The structure of the body is in essence a fluid/membrane continuum. The fluids of the body provide the stabilizing and cushioning forces that support the organs and other structures. Because of these hydrostatic forces, they can adapt instantly to the forces of compression. Peter Armitage, quoted above, likens this to cutting an apple: there is a crunchy, easy feel to cutting through the flesh of a healthy apple. However, when it is bruised the disrupted flesh has an altered fluid state, and so it responds differently to the compressive force of the knife. Similarly, when there is an altered fluid state in the body, as occurs in stasis, congestion or fibrosis the membranous wall becomes distorted. As a result, there is less capacity to adjust to the different levels of tension. The osteopath registers this as a dense 'feel' to the tissues.

The structural integrity and coherence of the body can be seen by the efficiency with which the body can maintain itself upright, or posture. The body maintains posture through constant checks and balances of tension in the ligaments and membranes and by minimal contraction and relaxation of muscles.

Posture

Posture is related to the spine, and its efficiency or balance is determined by an imaginary line through the body, termed the 'gravity line'. In an ideal posture, the head is well balanced above the sacrum. When looking at the erect body side on, an imaginary plumb line dropped from the ceiling should visibly pass through the ear, the shoulder, the middle of the third lumbar vertebra, the hip, in front of the sacrum, the middle of the knee and the ankle. This helps to assess the front to back curvatures and hence the forces of weight bearing on the body. The centre of gravity in the body is a theoretical point about two inches in front of the sacrum, when standing. Because it is so high from the ground, there is a greater potential for mobility and movement.

A good posture helps to maintain the internal environment of the body since it supports the function of the blood vessels and the position of the organs in their fluid compartments. A relatively symmetrical, well-balanced body is much more efficient than an asymmetrical one, since the body weight is evenly distributed with minimal energy requirements. But this is rare, and more often there is a lack of symmetry due to side dominance, so that the gravity line either shifts forwards or backwards. This causes an uneven distribution of body weight and so requires extra muscle energy to maintain an upright stance. You can check for yourself if your weight is falling centrally, forwards or backwards. Stand still and get someone to gently nudge your shoulder forwards. If you lose your balance, then you have an anterior weight-bearing posture so that the weight of your body is falling in front of the gravity line. If you lose your balance when you are nudged backwards from the shoulder, then you have a posterior weight-bearing posture.

In extremes of asymmetry there is a condition called scoliosis, which is an abnormal curvature of the spine and this can lead to the internal organs becoming compressed and twisted and therefore functioning less effectively.

Where the body is working from: the midline

Posture is related to the spine, but how we function and perceive ourselves is related to what the osteopath refers to as the 'midline'. When she looks at you and puts her hands on you, the osteopath feels the body as a whole unit, which is operating from a certain point of reference. How you feel about yourself and your perception of the world are essential to the proper functioning of the body. Think of how you feel when you are confident or when you hear good news – you feel expanded, energized, and your posture reflects this. Compare this to when you are down or unsure of yourself – the shoulders stoop and the posture sags, as does your energy. This reference point is where the body appears to be orientated, and is associated with the midline. This is neither visible nor is it fixed, but is really a sense of where the body organizes itself in order to function.

The midline originally appears as a groove when the embryo is just a mass of cells and later becomes our central nervous system. It forms the axis of orientation for the developing body. According to Dr James Jealous, the Breath of Life enters the body through the midline from where it generates the different forms of rhythms within the fluids, tissues and bioelectric fields. Once development is over, the midline remains as a palpable bioelectric line with the ability to shift automatically. This can be likened to the ever-moving electric spark that runs between the two ends of the filament in a light bulb. In the body, the two ends are the top and bottom ends of remnants of the very early nervous system of the embryo, and the electricity switching the bulb on can be likened to the Breath of Life. It is the axis of reference for the motions of the cerebrospinal fluid, the cranial and spinal membranes as well as the cranial bones.

Where we regard the centre of our being is pertinent not only to the psyche, but to the coping mechanisms of the body as well. In an ideal system, the midline and the gravity line superimpose. However, due to birth trauma and the stresses and strains of life, the midline will commonly shift to accommodate these challenges. This new axis becomes the line along which the body orients itself in order to function. When the body does not adapt well to this shift then an imbalance of its tissues occurs, often leading to a variety of symptoms. The osteopath's task is to re-establish the midline, and hence facilitate the healing processes to reorganize the body's structure and function.

The fulcrum

How you hold yourself in relation to space is a key factor for the osteopath when assessing the efficiency of body function. Think of how you feel when you've injured the shoulder. The tendency is to protect it by putting your hand over it and draw it closer into the body for comfort. The body adapts its functions from this point of hurt and even the neck bends towards it, so that the shoulder becomes the fulcrum around which the body works.

The fulcrum is a point around which the body as a whole, or any part of it, is functioning. It is a bit like the seesaw that goes up and down over a movable pivot, which can automatically shift to accommodate the weights sitting on either end. In other words, it is the area of stillness over which activity is occurring. The fulcrum is not a visible point but a sensation, and the osteopath feels this as the place where the body holds the greatest capacity to change its ability to function, or the 'site of potency'. It can be anywhere in the body: for instance, it may be at the cranial base, chest, diaphragm or the pelvis or even in the shoulder. It reveals the point from where the body tells its story. It is the point of comfort for that body and the osteopath will gauge the treatment around this fulcrum.

Again, in an ideal system, the whole body functions from a fulcrum that is within the midline. When there has been a traumatic event such as an accident or an emotional upset, the fulcrum deviates to accommodate the trauma, and may even be felt to be outside the body. People often describe this as not feeling grounded or centred and sayings such as 'I was beside myself' or 'I felt out of it' are apt in describing this externalizing of function. As a result, the body is not properly balanced and because it is not working efficiently, it uses excessive energy. The osteopath will often locate the point causing the body to be out of balance as a sense of inertia or 'pull' towards that area.

Body function and motion

When an osteopath talks about function, she is relating to the movement of and within the structure. In health, the body expresses its function through the movements of the framework and by the inherent motions that are present within its tissues. There are different types of tissues that make up the various structures of the body and so there are different types of motion expressed within them. These motions are related to the voluntary and involuntary mechanisms of the body.

Voluntary movement and mobility

When we think of movement, it is usually in terms of an activity brought about by the whole body, such as walking, talking, playing tennis or driving a car. This generally involves movements performed by the joints and muscles and this ability to move voluntarily gives us the freedom and skill to adapt to our environment.

To bring about this kind of body movement, one makes a conscious decision, as in playing the piano. This initiates a series of processes that activate nerves, muscles and other factors, which results in reading the music, playing the intricate composition on the keys and enjoying the melody.

In producing movements, we perform the activity through the voluntary mechanisms of the body. The movements that we initiate can either be 'active', such as that produced in flexing the arm, or 'passive' – for example, when the osteopath does it for you to assess the quality and range of movement in the elbow joint. Discomfort arising from restricted movement is often the reason behind a consultation. Postural defects, joint strains, disease, falls or accidents and scarring of the soft tissues may be contributing to such problems. In conditions that affect the joints, such as arthritis, movement is restricted both in the active and passive states.

Inherent motion

There is another kind of movement within the body. This is the motion of the internal organs and structures. Such motion, known as physiological motion, is continual, and we are rarely aware of it. It is expressed through the involuntary mechanisms of the body.

The internal organs express their function through inherent motions going on inside us at all times, regardless of our actions. These are the 'silent' structures, the internal machinery that quietly gets on with the business of sustaining our life. The essential physiological processes, such as clearance by the kidneys or exchange of gases in the lungs, continue whether we choose to play the piano or go to sleep.

There are many different inherent motions in the body, some of which are:

• Breathing of the lungs
• Cardiovascular rhythm of the heart and the blood vessels
• Peristalsis of the gut

Although we have little conscious control over these, we can greatly affect them through our moods and activities. When we need to adapt to a situation, such as running for a bus, the internal systems kick up a gear or two to give the energy and motion needed to catch the bus. Once the event is over, the gears soon drop back.

The adaptive mechanisms of the body allow us to respond to different situations, so when we ran for that bus, our breathing rate was increased. Equally, when we are tense or anxious, our gut might tighten and create rumblings. Having a dysfunctional relationship, poor eating and sleeping habits or smoking over a period of time may affect the cardiovascular rhythm. So, although the three functions listed are involuntary mechanisms, we can affect them somewhat.

Inherent motility

There is an even more subtle form of physiological inherent motion, since at the minute cellular level motion is also going on all the time. The body, over 70 per cent of which is water, is comprised of fluid-filled membranous sacs, which make up:

• The cells
• The organs within their capsules
• The fluid compartments within the fascias and the meningeal membranes

The tissues of the body are made up from cells and where there is cellular function, there is cellular motion. This type of inherent motion, which takes place throughout the system of fluids within the body, is known as 'motility'. The body of the developing embryo grows into the shape created by a fluid field, which means that the earliest inherent motion to be established is probably that of motility. The osteopath in working with primary respiration enlists it to influence the working of the body.

It is interesting that the breath is where involuntary and voluntary mechanisms meet and where the external and internal environments of the body interchange. And it is the case that through the conscious control of the muscles of breathing we can influence the inherent motion and therefore the function of the internal organs, as shown by practitioners of yoga.

The movements of the musculoskeletal system, the inherent motion of the internal organs and motility of the body fluids all influence each other. This becomes apparent as throughout life the body adapts to cope with long-term challenges, to respond to the cumulative stresses and strains of living. The natural tendency for motion in the cells is curtailed in response to injury, trauma or distress. If you about to be hit, the instinct is to withdraw into a tight ball; an injury will cause muscle spasm so that all its fibres contract, whilst an emotional upset causes us to feel withdrawn. The body's response to a challenge is to cause a contraction of its tissues, and as a result there is an altered fluid dynamic. The osteopath feels the results as an altered quality of motion within the internal structures and in the movements of the body framework. For example, with the condition of a 'frozen shoulder' there may be limited movement of the shoulder girdle, but there is still motion within its tissues. When there is a reduction in the inherent motion, there is potential for stasis and stagnation. The osteopath tunes in to the body's rhythms and is able to interpret and work towards amending any such abnormalities.

Chapter two

The body and primary respiration

The 'Breath of Life' is the spark, primarily, and not the breath of air. The breath of air is merely one of the material elements that the 'Breath of Life' utilizes in man's walk-about here on earth. In fact, the brain, the cerebrospinal fluid, the intracranial membranes, the physiological centres are merely secondary elements in that walk-about on earth.

Dr William Garner Sutherland

Osteopathy using primary respiration is often referred to as 'cranial' or 'craniosacral osteopathy', which could be taken to imply that it is only concerned with the head and pelvis. However, osteopathy is holistic medicine where the person is viewed as one unit, interacting with the environment. Although Sutherland described five anatomical and physiological factors that contribute towards the motions and functions of primary respiration, he did not partition these parameters, but always perceived the whole.

Physiological motion as an expression of primary respiration

The motions of primary respiration are described as being 'tide-like' and the osteopath feels them as very subtle but definite swelling and receding phases. They are the cumulative effects of the motions of the fluids, nervous tissues, membranes and bones. They are mainly felt at the head and sacrum, the two areas that may be considered as the hub of the mechanism, but can be felt throughout the body. These motions are quite different from the movements of breathing or the pulse of the heart, although all motions do influence each other. Like the other inherent motions of the body, those of primary respiration are biphasic in nature; that is to say, there are two 'halves' to the whole cycle and the motion exhibited in each is different.

The first phase is known as 'inhalation' and the second phase as 'exhalation'.

- During inhalation, the head feels as if it is expanding; midline structures of the body are felt to become short and fat, and simultaneously the bilateral structures are felt to roll outwards.
- During exhalation, the head feels as if it is contracting; the midline structures of the body are felt to become tall and thin, while the bilateral structures are simultaneously felt to roll inwards.

Dr Sutherland originally described five factors, each with its own motion, occurring both independently and simultaneously, as the 'primary respiratory mechanism'. These are:

- The cerebrospinal fluid (CSF)
- The brain and spinal cord (CNS)
- The cranial and spinal membranes or meninges
- The sacrum within the pelvic bones
- The individual cranial bones

When Sutherland originally described this anatomical/physiological complex in 1944, his studies were based on observation and self-experimentation. Since the mid-1980s, studies using the sensitivity of MRI techniques have verified brain and spinal cord motion as well as the fluctuating motion of the CSF.

These alternating rhythmic motions are considered by osteopaths to be an expression of the life force working within the whole body. The different types of tissues move to the Breath of Life, the instigator of all inherent motions. The interactions among the five factors may be likened to the mechanics of the heart. A comparison between the two might help to illustrate the point.

- The brain and the spinal cord are bathed in and contain the cerebrospinal fluid, just as the heart contains blood.
- Just as the blood has a pulse, the cerebrospinal fluid has a fluctuation.
- The brain and spinal cord are contained within fluid-filled membranous coverings known as the meninges, just as the heart is contained within its fluid-filled pericardial membranes.
- The movable bones of the cranium, the spinal vertebrae and the pelvis surround the brain, the spinal cord and its membranes, just as the heart with its vessels is enclosed within the movable bones of the chest.
- Just as the activity of the heart reaches the entire body with its motion felt at the arterial pulses, the motions of primary respiration also reach the entire body. The Breath of Life can be felt through all the fluids and membranes of the body: this takes us back to one of the basic principles of osteopathy, that the body is a single functional unit.

The primary respiratory mechanism

As we have seen, Sutherland referred to the five features as the 'primary respiratory mechanism' because the main control centres for the physiological processes of life (including breathing) are in the brain, which is of primary importance. The respiration aspect relates to the exchange of gases between the cells of the tissues and the fluids bathing them. It is the process by which cells can use nutritious substances and release waste material. These chemical reactions release energy, which the body uses for maintaining its processes. The inherent rhythmic motions are considered to be important to the homeostasis of the structure and function of the central nervous and hormonal systems as well as other aspects of function within the body physiology.

Each different type of tissue has its own response to primary respiration, felt as a distinct sensation particular to that tissue. Both Dr Still and Dr Sutherland considered the cerebrospinal fluid to be the most important element of the body and so we shall consider this aspect of the primary respiratory mechanism first.

The cerebrospinal fluid – its secretion and flow

The fluid compartments of the brain, known as ventricles, contain blood plexuses that secrete cerebrospinal fluid, CSF (see figure 2). It passes over the entire brain, its cranial nerves, the spinal cord and nerves. It then goes to the ganglia (a concentrated area of nerve tissue), connecting with the autonomic nervous system, before reaching the venous (blood) circulation. As it leaves the brain and spinal cord, a small amount eventually merges with the lymphatic circulation of the body. In this way, the CSF allows an interchange of substances between the blood and the lymphatic circulations.

The CSF is a highly refined product of the metabolism of food. Just as the blood transports nutrients, communication factors and other substances for the body, the CSF has similar functions within the central nervous system. The CSF interchanges its ions, neurotransmitters and nutritive factors between the following vital structures:

• Blood plexuses in the fluid ventricles of the brain
• Cells of the central, peripheral and autonomic nervous systems
• Hormones of the pituitary, pineal and hypothalamus glands

By working with the power or potency carried in the CSF, osteopathy can help to influence these interactions. In this way, fluid interchanges between the physiological centres at the area of the brain stem responsible for controlling the essential life processes, the autonomic centres in the brain, the hormonal glands and the special senses within the cranium (the eyes and ears) can be facilitated.

Working in this way is particularly useful where the body's tissues are exhausted. This is common after illnesses such as glandular fever, gastroenteritis and most post-viral syndromes, as well as autoimmune diseases

Figure 2 THE BASIC PARTS OF THE BRAIN AND THE FLOW
OF THE CEREBROSPINAL FLUID (CSF) IN THE CRANIUM

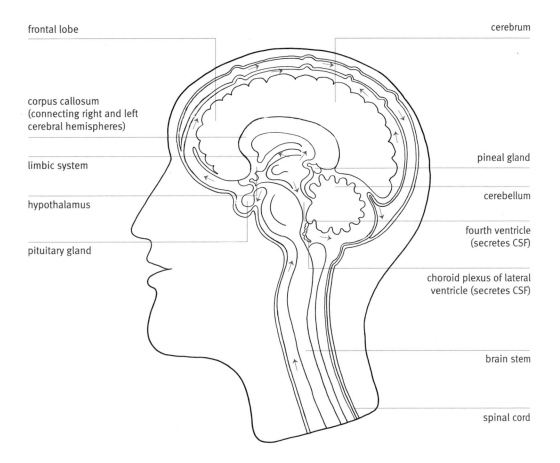

frontal lobe

cerebrum

corpus callosum
(connecting right and left
cerebral hemispheres)

pineal gland

limbic system

cerebellum

hypothalamus

fourth ventricle
(secretes CSF)

pituitary gland

choroid plexus of lateral
ventricle (secretes CSF)

brain stem

spinal cord

The different functions of the body and even emotions can be located in certain areas of the brain. The basic parts shown are:

- cerebrum – forming the main portion of the brain; the right and left hemispheres are connected by the corpus callosum
- cerebellum – dictates movements and co-ordination

- brain stem – connects the brain to the spinal cord
- limbic system – a group of structures related to smell, emotions and behaviour.

like rheumatoid arthritis. It is helpful where general tiredness is a symptom – often adolescents, for example, will seek help when they cannot study for lack of concentration and stamina. One of the objectives of working specifically with the fluid system and its lymphatic function is to allow the tissues to have fresh nourishment, which helps with vitality. Often in these cases, the fluid system has been sluggish over a long period of time, so there is poor nutrition of the body tissues. By working on fluid fluctuation and assisting movement within the fluid system, osteopathy can help to give a 'pick-me-up', and encourage the body's capacity to heal.

Another important function of the CSF is to provide buoyancy for the rather heavy brain. The average weight of the brain is 1500 grams (5 lb), but suspended in the CSF it exerts pressure equivalent to a weight of only about 50 grams (2 oz). The CSF is also important mechanically: if there were no cushioning, the brain would just bounce against the bony skull. Thanks to the wonderful self-protecting mechanisms of the CSF, any blows to the head move the whole brain so that the force of the blow is distributed evenly. So, where there is severe trauma to the head, the force of the hit will travel in the fluid medium to the opposite side of the skull and bruise that side of the brain, a feature known as 'contrecoup'. In general, the CSF protects the brain much better where there is a direct blow rather than where there is a large twisting or rotational force. If these forces are not resolved, they can affect the physiological motions of primary respiration and result in a variety of symptoms.

LUCY'S CHATTER

Lucy was a beautiful four-year-old girl who until six months ago had been known as a chatterbox. She had a lot going for her; intelligent and outgoing, she liked to be with people. That was before she had her fall. She had been sitting at breakfast when she lost her balance and fell backwards. She had fallen about two feet, hitting the right side of her head on the floor. Although there had been no brain damage or bleeding inside her head, since the accident she had spoken very few words and had become withdrawn. Her anxious parents had undertaken all the investigations possible in an effort to find out what was wrong but nothing had been discovered.

In the course of examination Lucy was found to have restricted primary respiratory motion throughout the body, but particularly noticeable at the speech area on the left side of her brain. This indicated that Lucy had become 'frozen' from the trauma of her fall. The poor motion through the speech centres of the brain was rather curious. When she fell, the blow to the head was on the side opposite to the speech areas. However, because there had been some twist as Lucy had fallen, the brain could not resolve the forces of strain and the speech areas were affected. Because she was constitutionally strong, once the fluidity of motion in this area and balance throughout her body had been restored she made a very quick recovery from the effects of the knock. She was chattering away again like her old self within weeks.

The blow to Lucy's head had affected both the fluctuation of the CSF and the inherent motion within the tissues of the brain. In addition the twist element of the fall was reflected within the cranial membranes, while the impact of the trauma was partly held in the cranial bones in the right side. So although the fall manifested as a change in behaviour and speech, where the brain needed particular attention, her total recovery in fact required a re-establishment of all the features of the primary respiratory mechanism.

The inherent motion of the brain and the spinal cord

Like all living tissues, the cells of the brain are capable of motility. The central nervous system (CNS) therefore has a mechanical action as well as its neurophysiological functions and its role as the co-ordinating system of the body.

Our knowledge of the brain is still in its infancy and we do not fully understand what each part of the brain does. Functions of consciousness, unconsciousness and emotions are still being unravelled. However, 'the map is not the territory' and often improving the motility of the CNS tissue will bring about a change in its overall function. With some conditions, there seems to be a typical pattern of reduced motion in certain areas; in autistics, for example, among other factors it is common to feel a limited motion through the frontal area of the brain. Encouraging the inherent motions seems to bring about an improvement to the overall functioning of the body unit. This is sometimes witnessed as a change in personality or behaviour.

After Lucy had her fall, the part of the brain where motion felt reduced was in the area that is related to speech. This was not seen in any previous investigations because most methods used catch the body and brain parts in a still frame. It would be like trying to use an X-ray to catch the motion of breath through the lungs. The inherent motion of the brain is extremely subtle but has a profound influence.

Movement of the cranial bones

The different bones of the cranium are loosely bonded and can therefore accommodate the inherent motions of the brain, spinal cord and its fluid. They almost seem to go for a ride on these structures, by virtue of the attachments of the meninges and the dynamics of the fluids.

The bones of the cranium

The cranium is made up of some 26 different bones. Just as there are movements between the individual vertebrae of the spine, so too there are micro-movements between the bones of the head and face. Where each bone fits into the other, there is a specialized joint called a suture that allows for motion between them. (See figure 3.)

As well as being able to articulate with each other, living bones are pliable. They too contain fluid. They respond to the other components of the primary respiratory mechanism as well as to the external forces of compression from weight and gravity. This is particularly significant in babies, where pliability and

Figure 3 THE BONES OF THE CRANIUM
           side view

suture or joint between
movable cranial bones

parietal bone   frontal bone

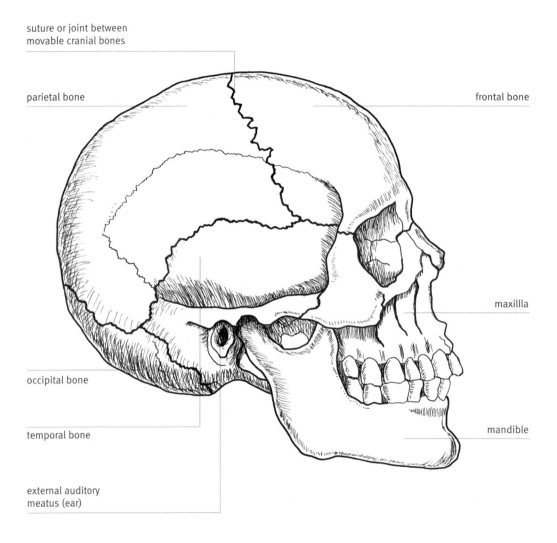

                                                                   maxillla

occipital bone

                                                                   mandible

temporal bone

external auditory
meatus (ear)

articular mobility of the cranium enables the baby to pass through the birth canal and accommodate the forces of birth.

Mobility and pliability of the cranial bones are important for full expression of the cranium's underlying structures, the CNS and CSF. Imagine a wooden box containing, say, mangos. If there is a distortion in the shape of the box, it will create pressure on the mangos directly under it. Where there is a restriction or distortion of any of the cranial bones, the inherent motion is inhibited and this creates an area of dysfunction. This may arise directly from being hit on the head or from birth strain, or indirectly from, for example, a fall on the bottom.

The bones at the cranial base

When there is a restriction to the movements between the cranial bones, there are many and varied symptoms displayed by the body. This is in part because there are holes or 'foramina' between the cranial bones for blood vessels and nerves leaving and entering the cranial cavity (see figure 4). The effects of restrictions of the cranial sutures are very similar to those of the vertebral joints, in the sense that they affect the nerve and blood supplies. Some significant points are that:

- Any bony restrictions inhibit the motions of the primary respiration.
- There will be a mechanical influence on the flow of blood carrying oxygen and nutrients to the brain and head.
- Major nerves exit the cranial base through the foramina between the bones, and bony restrictions may affect the cranial nerves locally.
- The jaw and teeth may be affected, as may the function of the special senses, for example the eyes through the bones making up the orbits; the ears through the bones that house them; and the bones making up the sinuses and the nose.

IRENE'S FACE ACHE
Irene had to come back early from her holiday in Scotland. She had found the weather particularly windy, although her husband thought it was perfectly normal. Each time the wind brushed against her face, she suffered intense pain in her teeth. Before she went on holiday she had had occasional aches in the side of her face, with odd tingling sensations. Her teeth, although in good working condition, were now sensitive to cold, hot foods and sweets. She arrived saying this was the worst pain she had ever known.

As I examined her, there was a lot of compression in the area of the jaw and particularly at the cranial base. She seemed 'stuck' here. She revealed that she had suffered on and off from sinusitis and this made the facial pain much worse. She also had a fair bit of dental work with heavy fillings over many years. Having carefully checked for motion in each part of the head and face, it was clear to me that the left temporal bone was not moving properly and the membranes attached to it were strained. As a result the ganglion from the cranial (the trigeminal) nerve that is situated here was affected. The poor lady was suffering from irritation of this nerve,

Figure 4 THE BONES AT THE CRANIAL BASE
Seen from under the cranium

hypoglossal canal beneath condylar part of the occipital bone for the twelfth (hypoglossal) nerve and meningeal artery (tongue muscles)

occipital bone at the back of the head

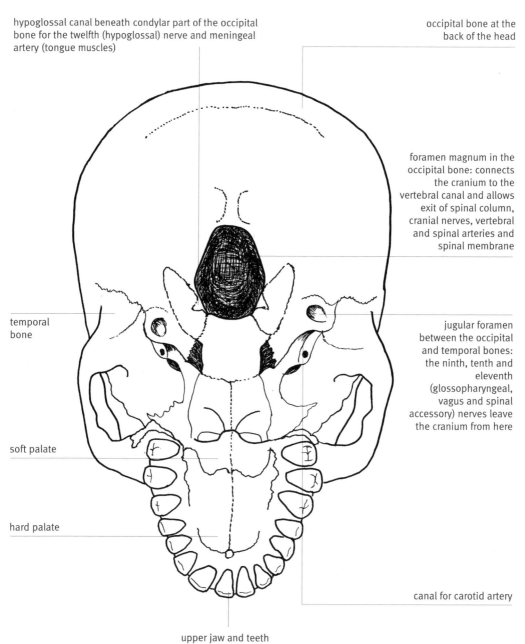

foramen magnum in the occipital bone: connects the cranium to the vertebral canal and allows exit of spinal column, cranial nerves, vertebral and spinal arteries and spinal membrane

temporal bone

jugular foramen between the occipital and temporal bones: the ninth, tenth and eleventh (glossopharyngeal, vagus and spinal accessory) nerves leave the cranium from here

soft palate

hard palate

canal for carotid artery

upper jaw and teeth

known as 'trigeminal neuralgia', whose origin may well have been from the bones at the cranial base getting jammed through repeated dental trauma. Once the bony and membranous functions were restored through subtle manipulations, and the rest of the head and neck was balanced in relation to this, Irene's symptoms gradually began to subside. Now she just returns for some 'facial maintenance' when she thinks she is going to get pain, or has sensitive teeth. This usually occurs when she is feeling tense or overwhelmed.

The cranial membranes

The cranial membranes form pleats and at certain points attach into the movable bones of the cranium, so that the cavity is separated into four quadrants. These partition the right and left hemispheres of the brain from the right and left cerebellar lobes. (See figure 5.)

Tension in the membranes

The balance of tension within the body and its membranes is critical for structural integration and coherence. The cranial and spinal membranes provide both a tensional mechanism for moving the cranial bones and the sacrum, as well as a guiding and restraining action. The dural meningeal membranes of the brain and the spinal cord connect the cranium to the sacrum. Within the cranium, the dural membrane folds back on itself, forming two pleats that separate the brain into right and left halves and front and back parts. At certain key areas it attaches to the movable bones of the cranium. On exiting the cranium it attaches at the second vertebra of the neck, just like hooks holding up a curtain. This 'dural curtain' traverses the whole length of the spine freely while still covering and protecting the spinal cord and its nerves, finally hooking into the base of the spine and the sacrum.

The dural curtain is continuous and is structurally important in many ways. It separates the brain into four quadrants, forms a window for the labyrinth of the ears, and ensheathes the cranial nerves. It also functions as a shock and stress absorber for the brain and spinal cord. Mechanically, the dural curtain links the cranium with the sacrum so that whatever is happening at the top can be felt at the bottom, and vice versa, in much the same way that pulling on the bottom of the shirt sleeve will be felt as tension at the shoulder. Such monitoring is possible because of the degree of tension created in this firm but elastic membrane, where tension functions in a delicate state of balance and equilibrium. The normal tension may be altered through a wide variety of factors, such as bony restrictions, surgical adhesions, dehydration through illness, and physical or emotional trauma. Membranes are also vulnerable to forces of distortion from stressful situations, such as breaks or falls. Because they line the brain like a skin and are also attached to bones, the membranes act as a medium through which forces of stress may be transmitted to and from the brain. The tensions created within membranes by an illness, stress or injury

Figure 5 THE PLEATS OF THE DURAL CRANIAL MEMBRANE
Bone cut away to show cranial membrane and its pleats.

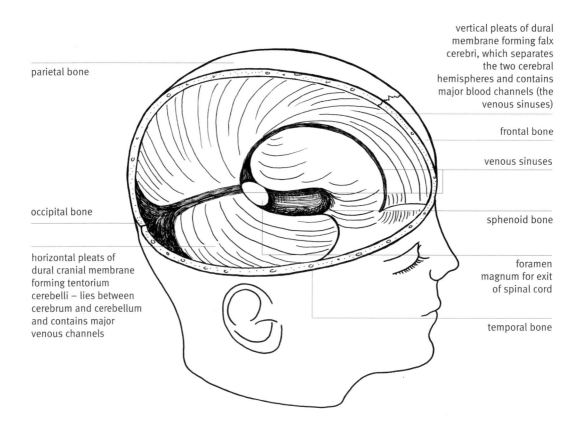

vertical pleats of dural membrane forming falx cerebri, which separates the two cerebral hemispheres and contains major blood channels (the venous sinuses)

parietal bone

frontal bone

venous sinuses

occipital bone

sphenoid bone

horizontal pleats of dural cranial membrane forming tentorium cerebelli – lies between cerebrum and cerebellum and contains major venous channels

foramen magnum for exit of spinal cord

temporal bone

are known as the 'lesion pattern' and can be very strong. Unless they are released, they hold this strain pattern even though it might have occurred a very long time ago. In doing so, the excessive tension inhibits the expression of primary respiration, and this is reflected throughout the body.

MAX'S BEGINNING

Let us return to Julie and her son Max, whom I introduced right at the beginning of the book. Stuart had greatly eased Max's discomfort merely by placing his hands on the bottom. What happened? Max had been irritable and fractious for all his short life and yet the symptoms eased within minutes of our holding the sacrum and pelvis. Why?

Max's problem was related to his birth. As he tried to come out of the birth canal, his head had got stuck. Because the bones of the baby's skull are rather soft and pliable they can usually adjust to this situation without any great difficulty. In Max's case, however, the greatest stress had been to the membranes lining the bones of the skull. As the head got stuck, the cranial bones overlapped causing the skull to change its shape so that it could come through the birth canal. This distortion in the bones had to be checked by reciprocal tension in the membranes, which they recorded as stress. But long after his birth, Max's body could not resolve this tension. Because they also act as a 'skin' covering for the brain, the excessive tension in the membranes must also have given poor Max a huge headache and made him understandably irritable. So naturally he would not let me anywhere near his head.

The only way to release the stress in the membranes was from the sacrum, the other end of the circuit. Using the sacrum as a lever to take the slack off the membranes, the tension at the cranium was gently unwound. In this way the stress in Max's system was subtly and yet profoundly eased; this was noticeable through the changes in breathing pattern, the colour of the face and the fact that he just dropped off to sleep.

Involuntary mobility of the sacrum at the pelvis

As we have seen, the sacrum and the coccyx complete the reciprocal tensional circuit by providing for lower attachments to the dural curtain. The sacrum sits in the pelvis suspended between its two bones by very strong ligaments, like ropes, providing both stability and mobility. The sacrum also provides a weight bearing function by dispersing the compressive forces throughout the continual tensional network since it gives anchorage for the dural curtain. It also carries and transports nerves from the lower part of the spinal cord. This mean that reduced motion in the sacrum can also have an effect on the structures supplied by these nerves.

Like the cranial bones, the sacrum is not moved by muscles, but by the tension within the spinal membranes attached to it and therefore it displays the movements of primary respiration. Because of the tensional effects, any dysfunctional stress patterns in the sacrum may give symptoms in the head.

Equally, tensions within the membranes at the cranium may inhibit the motions of the sacrum (see figure 6).

ELIZABETH'S HEADACHE

Elizabeth had been undergoing dental work. But, because she had constant head pain, she could not cope with the teeth restorations. Her dentist, who got tired of her complaining, finally referred her to the clinic. She had no other symptoms – just a constant ache all over her head, which was getting worse. She was taking a lot of painkillers to get some relief but was now feeling tired, vulnerable and irritable. The headaches started when she fell on her bottom as she took the quicker route down the stairs. At the time she was only slightly shaken and since the fall had been minor she had not linked it to the headaches.

I examined her neck, shoulders and the head, but found nothing of significance. However, when placing my hand at the sacrum, I found it to be crammed within the pelvis, which limited its inherent motions. Most of the force from the fall had wedged the sacrum within the pelvic bones, whilst the rest had travelled up the spine into the cranium where the upper part of the dural membrane curtain 'hooks' in. Because of this, the bones of the cranial base had become held in a position that matched the force and direction of the fall on the bottom. Her treatment merely required disengaging the sacrum from its wedged position in the pelvis, realigning the coccyx and unwinding the curtain. This allowed the cranial base to become free and re-engage its motions freely. As the system rebalanced, Elizabeth's headaches began to diminish and finally subside.

It is interesting to note that both Max and Elizabeth had suffered with head problems that were released from the sacrum. They had, however, acquired their problems for different reasons. Max's head had got stuck *en route*, while it was Elizabeth's sacrum that was stuck. In both cases, the cranial mechanics were disturbed due to the membranous connections between the sacrum and the cranium, which had in turn disturbed the fluid hydraulics. In Max's case, the sacrum was free to move and so this was used as a lever to influence the cranial motion, while in Elizabeth's case the sacrum itself needed to be freed.

In the above examples, each anatomical and physiological aspect of the primary respiratory mechanism has been described separately to illustrate its contribution to ill heath. In reality, however, it is difficult to distinguish between them, and all aspects occur simultaneously.

The transverse planes: diaphragms

Relevant factors are the sheets of muscles and ligaments that form transverse planes for the body: these are known as diaphragms. They separate the body into four compartments, the cranium, the chest, the abdomen and the pelvis. While they support and interconnect the internal organs, through the tensional network they also affect the function of the organs contained in the compartments above and below.

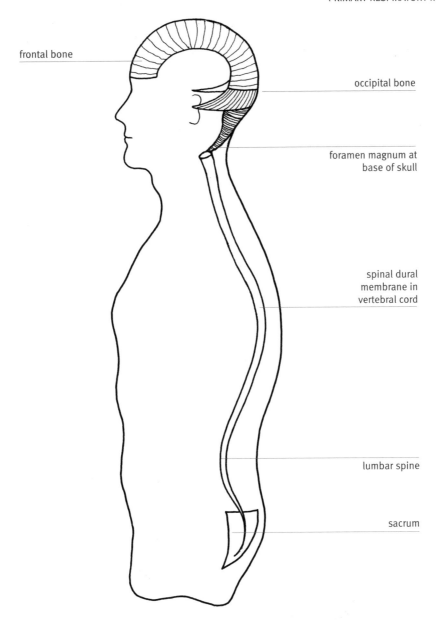

frontal bone

occipital bone

foramen magnum at
base of skull

spinal dural
membrane in
vertebral cord

lumbar spine

sacrum

The coverings of the brain and spinal cord are the three meningeal membranes. The inner two are the pia and arachnoid, between which the CSF flows. These form a 'skin' for the central nervous system, while the outermost layer is dura, which is attached at various points to the movable bones of the skull, to the top of the spine , and in the lower lumbar spine and sacrum.

Because of these connections, a tension mechanism is created in the membranes which acts with the fluid system so that motions in the cranium can also be felt in the sacrum, and vice versa. The fluid nature of the body and its membranous interconnections means that these inherent motions can be felt throughout the body.

The most familiar of these is the thoracic diaphragm found in the middle of the body. This big muscle divides the body into the thorax above and the abdomen below. Its rhythmic breathing motions gently massage the heart and lungs above and the stomach, intestines, liver and other structures just below it. The cranial diaphragm is made from the meningeal membranes and its functions have been described above. The ligaments and soft tissues attaching into the sacrum and coccyx form the pelvic floor or diaphragm. The integrity of this will have a bearing on the urinary and reproductive structures of the pelvic cavity. The importance of the diaphragms is that each has its own rhythmic motion. The movement at the cranial diaphragm is involuntary and that of the pelvic diaphragm is synchronous with it. Although the rhythm of the thoracic diaphragm in breathing is separate, each one influences the others.

The fascias of the body are normally vertically orientated, and permit the natural sliding and gliding motions of the internal organs such as the liver, which normally moves in response to body movements. On the other hand the diaphragms – that is, the cranial membranes, the thoracic diaphragm and the pelvic floor – are orientated horizontally. This means that any strain within the diaphragms, such as may occur after a fall or accident, can inflict a dragging force on the fascial planes and so indirectly interfere with the natural gliding motions of the internal organs and primary respiration.

Why primary respiration is important to health

Osteopaths using primary respiration regard it as an important anatomical and physiological complex that affects health in different ways. In ill health, the quality of the primary respiration is altered; when reinstated, it helps to restore body physiology. Primary respiration influences and is in turn influenced by:

• The vascular or circulatory system
• The nervous system
• The musculoskeletal system
• The lymphatic system
• The respiratory system
• The hormonal or endocrine system

Some specific physiological mechanisms are:

Blood and nutrition (See figures 4 and 5.)

Blood vessels enter and leave the brain via small openings or foramina between the bones, and the membranes that line the cranium contain major veins (venous sinuses). Therefore the movements of the cranial bones can affect the flow of blood and substances carried to and from the brain.

Impeded venous and lymphatic drainage is an important cause of stasis and congestion within the body. Excessive tension in the membranes and restricted mobility of the cranial bones alters the drainage mechanisms in the cranium. By improving these, the flow of oxygen and nutrients to the brain can be enhanced.

Homeostatic function (See figure 2.)

At the base of the cranium and top of the neck lies an area of the brain referred to as the 'magic inch'. It contains the homeostatic control centres for the regulation of the heart rate, blood pressure, swallowing, breathing, talking and vomiting.

Because this area of the brain stem is indirectly influenced by the mechanics of the cranial bones and the attached dural membranes, by working here the osteopath can influence most of the metabolic and regulatory functions of the body. Helping with panic attacks and the regulation of breathing in an asthma attack are two examples of 'quick fixes' that are possible. Naturally, people suffering from these conditions will have other problems, which are also supported.

Cranial nerves (See figure 4.)

Membranes within the cranium cover the cranial nerves, and like blood vessels they too leave the cranium through various foramina. So any bony restrictions, membranous tension or venous congestion may lead to their irritation. Since the cranial nerves supply so much, all sorts of problems can arise. Difficulty in suckling or swallowing in a newborn due to irritation of the twelfth nerve and the type of trigeminal neuralgia we saw with Irene are just two conditions that can be helped by freeing the nerves within the cranium.

Hormonal or endocrine function (See figure 14.)

The pituitary and pineal glands within the cranium affect the function of other glands in the body. When there are mechanical distortions of the bones, membranes or fluids, they can result in associated chemical and electrical imbalances that release stress-producing factors. The hypothalamus, within the cranium, controls the autonomic nerves and glands within the body. If its function is affected then physical or emotional trauma can make a greater impact than the trauma would warrant and this can lead to ill health, emotional conflict or tension. Rebalancing the area that mediates the nervous-hormonal pathways can counteract such stress-producing factors.

Immune function

Primary respiration aids in immune function since the lymphatic fluids partake in the absorption of CSF. This encourages 'lymphatic drainage' through the lymphatic chain of the body, so supporting its immune function. In addition, there is 'chatter' between the hypothalamus and the pituitary axis in the brain and the cells of the immune system, so that stress-producing factors released from the brain affect the immune function.

The osteopath will be reading all aspects of primary respiration so as to assess the body on different levels. Which is where we came in at the beginning of the chapter. If we have a fall, an infection or an emotional trauma, the body responds by making sure that we do not go out of kilter. But although a particular area might be hurt, the response to the injury takes place within the entire body.

Chapter three

Finding the cause of discomfort

To find health should be the object of the doctor. Anyone can find disease.

Dr Andrew Taylor Still, *The Philosophy and Mechanical Principles of Osteopathy*

Mrs Brown had been suffering with a horribly painful knee for about three months and repeatedly visited her general practitioner. Finally, to satisfy her questions about her deteriorating state, he advised her that she had arthritis, a condition of wear and tear. She naturally asked why this had occurred. He replied that it was due to her age. To this she retorted, through sheer frustration, 'Well, the other knee is the same age – why doesn't that one bother me?'

Why indeed? The arthritis of the knee was the effect of a breakdown in the function of the joint. The puzzle lay in finding why her body had brought that knee (as opposed to the other one) to its current painful, inflamed state.

In searching for the cause of discomfort, we are seeking a diagnosis. This is more than just giving a label to a set of signs and symptoms presented to us by the patient. To be able to describe a condition, such as a 'bursitis resulting in a frozen shoulder', and then treat only the anatomical and physiological aspects, is just the beginning of the healing process. Diagnosis lies in understanding the relationship of the whole body to the area in trouble. Often this is not revealed in a single session. Deep underlying factors may have been long forgotten by the mind but are filed away, to be dealt with later by the body.

The body maintains its functions through constant complicated checks and balances of its co-ordinated biochemical, bioelectrical and biomechanical processes. Where most systems of medicine are concerned with the biochemical cause of disease, osteopathy searches for bio-mechanical and biodynamic dysfunctions as well. When the body expresses movement and motion freely, it is more able to function and repair itself from disease. But it is also the case that mechanical stress factors play a big part in altering tissue chemistry.

The osteopath's methods are very simple and yet require a high degree of skill and experience. The osteopath employs the usual medical investigation procedures when required, but is not solely reliant on them; the primary tools of the trade are touch and observation. The skill of osteopathy lies in being able to feel and recognize normal function from altered function and to 'read' the comparative quality of the tissues in the body.

The osteopath develops particular qualities of perception: she will be watching to see how you relate to the external surroundings as well as what is happening internally. Posture and carriage reveal the structural integrity of the body and the psyche, while any changes to the skin give clues to the internal processes. The facial and body expression as well as a sense of the body field is also acknowledged. An osteopath observes not only with the eyes but with her whole being.

The osteopathic touch: palpation, perception and purpose

All professions have a tool with which they work, and the osteopath is no exception. She has learned a particular sense of touch. Just as the taste buds of the wine taster can differentiate between the different vintages of wine, so too can the touch of an osteopath detect areas of normal and altered function in the body.

Touch can mean many things and be interpreted in just as many ways – a mother's reassuring touch, the caress of a lover, or a touch that feels invasive when not wanted. A touch that has too much pressure hurts, while touch without attention will give little feedback. The osteopathic touch is sensitive, light, but definite.

The way the osteopath uses her hands is special. They are like satellite dishes that receive information from the body, feeling for different tissue tensions and their quality, for the body's inherent rhythmic motions or for motion that is 'frozen'. It is not just a passive process where the osteopath waits and sees. The hands receive information, which is felt as micro-movements and tensions within the body. This is then amplified by applying very subtle movement and pressure so that the information can be recorded and actively processed.

Touch is used to assess what is happening in the body at any level, superficial or deep. Essentially, the body is made up of fluid-containing tissues of varying densities. At the superficial level, changes in the skin are evident in terms of texture, colour, lumps and bumps or heat and sweatiness. Within the deeper structures, changes in fluidity, elasticity and tension can also be perceived as indicators of health or strain.

Here is an account of the tissue structures of the body and their relative densities:

Heavy density	Medium density	Light density	Very light density
Hard tissues:	Soft tissues:	Membranes:	Fluids:
Bone	Muscle	Dura	CSF
Cartilage	Fascia		Lymph
	Ligaments		Blood

There is a different feel to tissues that are in or out of balance, healthy or sick, normal or abnormal in each person. In diagnosis and treatment, the osteopath uses touch to detect very minute and subtle changes within the body's environment and physiology. In fact, trained hands can estimate the temperature of the body, blood pressure and the virulence of a viral infection to quite a marked degree. Feeling for the tissue quality, tone and the anatomic and physiological relationships enables the osteopath to make a fairly accurate diagnosis. When the osteopath is feeling the motion of primary respiration, she is using the same mechanisms as those used by the blind to gauge the position of the body in the dark, known as the 'proprioceptive system'. We know these to be absolutely reliable and sensitive systems within us and depend on them implicitly in the dark. It is through this same means that the osteopath's hands can sense what is happening in the body.

The search for discomfort

In searching for the cause of discomfort, osteopathy is concerned with more than just the identification and treatment of disease: the person with the disease is as important as the disease with which the person is afflicted. The search therefore begins with careful questioning and listening to a detailed history of the person concerned. A physical examination follows when the osteopath will be observing and listening to the body.

The first objective is to examine the usual state of tissues of the person in discomfort. Only when what is 'normal' for that individual at that particular time in their life has been established is it possible to understand and treat the 'abnormal'. Every condition has an explanation. For the osteopath, searching for the roots of the presenting symptom picture is of vital importance in understanding how the condition has come about in that person.

When you first visit your osteopath, the search begins almost at an unconscious level even before beginning the formal examination. She will start her assessment as you walk in, noting how you hold yourself, which way you lean, body actions and how you sit down, cluing in on how you function even before you've discussed the problem.

Questions asked

Building up a picture of the patient means asking for the life story. The osteopath may begin with the immediate problems, precipitating factors, how it started, the progression and any other difficulties. She will ask about any accidents, injuries, hospitalization, vaccinations, or any difficult periods. Details of current or past medications, the nature of present or any previous long-standing occupations and leisure activities are asked for. Pregnancies, allergies, eye or ear problems and any health issues as well as dental work and eating habits are also taken into account. You will even be asked for your birth history and childhood illnesses. Any deviations from the usual patterns such as sleeping habits, weight changes, hair loss, state of skin and fingernails, times of the day when hungry or tired and night sweats are all clues as to how the body is functioning.

What?

Since discomfort can mean a number of things to people, my opening question is usually 'How can I help you?' The answer enables me to understand how the person perceives their own condition. Pain is the commonest reason for people seeking help from an osteopath, but there may be other problems, such as restricted mobility within one or more parts of the body. These may be associated with other symptoms such as pins and needles or a loss of sensation or strength in one or both limbs. Feeling 'out of sorts' or being generally unwell is another reason why people seek help.

With children discomfort is more difficult to identify. Parents generally report that their child is suffering from a diagnosed condition such as asthma, colic, glue ear or is generally not doing well at school or a number of other behavioural problems.

Where?

As well as describing in words where the pain or discomfort is, the patient is asked to point to the area of discomfort and how far it spreads. Any associated phenomena, such as pain in the neck at the same time as getting a migraine, for example, are also located.

How?

Finding out how the problem arose helps the osteopath to assess the body's mechanisms of adaptation. She will also take into account how the body is used both at work and at home so that overall stresses and strains can be ascertained. In Mrs Brown's case, the knee pain had only bothered her during the last few months, and had appeared for no apparent reason. But as I watched her walking, I noticed that she seemed to lean more on the affected leg. She herself had not noticed this tendency, but when probed remembered that as a young woman she had fallen from her horse and landed on the opposite side to the offending knee. At the time she suffered with a painful 'hip' for some months, but was fine after a while.

When the order of events was put together, it became clear that the forces leading to discomfort in the right knee had been established a long time ago. The fall had bruised the left side of the pelvis so that while walking she favoured the opposite side, which added to the weight-bearing forces on this knee. This 'pattern' of a left-sided fall had been recorded in her tissues, which led her to maintain the lean. Over a period of time, this stress would naturally lead to excessive wear and tear or 'arthritis' due to the uneven forces of compression and weight bearing.

When?

Knowing how long the problem has been there will help to assess the state or quality of the tissues. A new injury, for example, means that recently bruised tissues are in a state of inflammation, and the degree of pain is more intense. In addition, although there are immediate local effects, the rest of the body has not yet had a chance to work itself around the area of discomfort. If, on the other hand, the problem has been there for some time, the rest of the body has had a while to adapt or 'compensate' in an attempt to maintain the normal functioning.

In Mrs Brown's case, the initial fall on to the pelvis caused the back muscles to tighten up in order to protect it. Over a period of time this led to an imbalance in the pelvis and an unequal pull of the leg muscles. At the same time, the extra weight-bearing forces meant the muscles could not relax and so they became ropey, losing elasticity at a faster rate than normal. The breakdown in function meant the right knee was subject to extra wear and tear.

Why?

When seeking the cause of discomfort, the main question is, why has this particular patient presented at this particular time with this particular problem? What caused this body to become so out of balance as to make this person seek help now? The body has undergone a series of postural, emotional, physical and psychological stresses long before we take notice on a conscious level. It seems that the body uses the way we respond to pain as a strategy to gain our attention.

In the example we've been looking at, why did the body finally lose its structural integrity or its ability to compensate, so that the knee became sufficiently painful for the lady to seek help? When walking, she had been leaning too heavily on the right knee, placing even greater stress on a vulnerable area. She could to a great extent put up with the pain, but the real reason why she had presented at this time was that she could no longer walk very far with her husband, which saddened her. This sense of loss was perhaps as significant as the physical pain in bringing Mrs Brown to her consultation.

The examination

Once the osteopath is satisfied that the story fits with the symptom picture, she will need to verify it through examining the body. This starts with an overall functional assessment of the body, followed by that of specific parts. Through observation and palpation, she reaches a diagnosis, but may continue to ask various questions as she examines you.

Most osteopaths have a routine they follow, except of course when examining children, who dictate that you fit around their needs! This is also true of those in intense pain or the very sick. This approximate (by no means exhaustive) routine, which can be varied according to circumstances, is outlined below:

Observation

- Perception of the person, poise, the relationship of the body in space and how the story is told.
- Standing examination – posture, integrity of the body, any twitches or tremors.
- Structural asymmetries, leans or twists in the body, leg lengths, relationship of limbs to the pelvis, shoulder girdles and the spine.
- Skin colour, texture, lumps, bumps, sweatiness, unusual hair patches or scarring.
- Performance of simple 'active' movements – bending forwards, backwards and so on to check for range, quality, lean and ease of movements performed. Special tests for different functions such as weight-bearing, for example at the hip.
- Sitting examination – as above.

Palpation

- Lying down, on either side or on the back or front. Palpation of specific areas for texture and integrity of surrounding soft tissues.
- Testing for range, quality of the gross movements of the spinal and peripheral joints by introducing 'passive' motion and mobility tests – any areas of restricted or too much movement, impaction or strain are indicative of dysfunction and mechanical breakdown at this level. This task may also be performed whilst sitting.
- Specific clinical examinations: leg-raising test, reflexes, muscle strength, blood pressure, listening to chest or other tests as required.
- Examination using primary respiration and inherent motion.

Palpation of inherent motion

When the osteopath puts her hands on the body, she is assessing the tissues to see how the body is working and how it has responded to previous problems. Osteopathy regards motion to be the gauge for healthy and sick tissues. The osteopath feels the efficiency with which tissues perform their function through the inherent rhythmic motion of primary respiration. Healthy tissues have a free and easy quality, which feels as if the cells themselves are breathing in and out – expanding and contracting without effort. On the other hand, sick tissues express lesser yet more strenuous motion, with a poor expansion and contraction – they feel weary. The osteopath assesses the qualitative feel of the tissues and how this is reflected in terms of fluidity, compression or tightness.

The osteopath tunes in to the overall pattern of body function and feels for the normal motions within the tissues. These usually become altered in ill health, and exaggerated breathing or suckling in babies can often help the osteopath to feel them more efficiently.

The different aspects of primary respiration in health are expressed around the central axis of the body, but tend to become displaced in ill health so the body is using extra energy to retain its sense of balance. In making a diagnosis using primary respiration, the osteopath is assessing motion within all the tissues of the body, including the bones, the membranes and the fluids.

When feeling the bones, the osteopath senses joint movement or a lack of it in the cranial sutures, whose inherent motion is dictated by the tension in the membranes. She also feels for the resilience or plasticity within the bone tissues. Each bone is capable of different movements such as flexion, extension and so on. When the osteopath induces a particular movement, the tissues reveal how far or how little they like to go in that direction. The membranes and the CSF carry out the slow, gentle change of position and this helps to find the position of ease or restriction in an area of the body. By working out the way the tissues like to be, the patterns of function can be named and defined. Strain patterns may be complex. Prolonged tension in the membranes, for example, becomes more damaging when it is unevenly distributed. This often becomes evident in the muscles attached to the outside of the skull. Internally, it is present in such structures as the fascia which sheaths the blood vessels and nerves as they exit the skull.

In examining the motions of primary respiration, the osteopath may have a routine, such as the one below, that she follows. Again this is by no means exhaustive. She looks for:

- A sense of an overall fulcrum of the body: the point from where the body is functioning, whether it is central to the body, through its gravity point or somewhere else.
- Areas of restricted rhythmic motion and membranes under strain as compared with motion in an area that is normal.
- The movements of the cranial bones in relation to each other in response to a given direction. For example, the cranium may seem to expand and rotate more on one side than the other. The bones are also assessed for pliability.
- By adding a gentle nudge, the osteopath may match the compression felt in the tissues to receive feedback, similar to checking the ripeness of a fruit. This exaggerates the pattern within the membranes or the fluids, so revealing the body's patterns for previous injury or disease.
- The movement within the sacrum and its relationship to the cranial and spinal membranes and the rest of the body.
- Patterns of motion in the arms and legs or other specific areas of the body.

The osteopath uses the above features to assess the motion of primary respiration and to uncover the cause of discomfort. Patterns of stress and strain are felt as tension or fixed points within the tissues of the body, which can be assessed by their symmetry, amplitude and quality of motion, described below.

Symmetry

As the alternate rhythmic motion of primary respiration is felt all over the body, so there is symmetry. When there is a problem in an area of the body, such as the knee, the rhythm will be felt but its intensity will differ from that of the other side.

Total symmetry is usually felt when there are no problems and is occasionally witnessed in newborn or very young babies. Lack of symmetry indicates an area of dysfunction and some reasons for this are joint dysfunction, inflammation, poor motility in the organs and internal structures, trauma or surgical scarring. Motion here is different or difficult to feel when compared to the other side. This is a good prognosticator. If, after treatment, motion is the same as the other side then the capacity for change within the body is good. On the other hand, if the asymmetry returns within the next session, then the capacity to hold a change is poor and progress may well be slow.

Amplitude

When the osteopath places her hands on either side of the head, in the inhalation phase of primary respiration, it feels as if it is expanding. The term amplitude relates to the maximum extent or breadth of the motion of expansion, before moving into the phase of exhalation and contraction of the head. Checking amplitude is another useful diagnostic tool. In good health the amplitude feels wide, reflective of the body's vitality or ability to cope and recover from a stressful situation. It may be lessened after an emotional trauma, chronic fatigue or other debilitating condition. This is suggestive of reduced vitality and ability to cope with future exposure to infection, distress or physical trauma and recovery may also be slower than expected.

Quality

This is the ease with which the body can express the inherent motions of primary respiration: Becker describes it as the 'voltage'. The body has a power within it, which is reflected in the quality of its tissues. A higher voltage means a greater capacity for achieving wellbeing, while a poor quality indicates a slower capacity. This is especially useful to bear in mind in treatment, since the higher voltage patient will be able to handle big changes. Where the lower voltage patient is concerned, the osteopath has to treat just enough and be prepared for a slower recovery, otherwise the tissues will get exhausted.

The quality of a person's tissues is influenced by health, nutrition, environment and genetics. Any disease processes, trauma or emotional stress will also modify them, as will osteopathy. The tissues making up the anatomy of the body are basically bone, soft tissues and fluids. The inherent motion of each type of tissue has its own peculiar feel so that motion through a bony area will be different from that within a membranous or fluid area in the same person. What is 'normal' tissue will also vary from person to person. The muscle tone of an athlete, for example, is quite different from that of a sumo wrestler of the same age. Equally, the feel of tissues alters with age so that the tissues of a baby are quite different from those of an adolescent or older person. The resilience, resistance and texture of each person are variable so that not all normal tissues are the same: it is an individual matter.

Also, the quality of tissues differs in health and ill health. When working with primary respiration, the osteopath feels dysfunction within the different tissues as variations in tension, motion and vitality. In the membranes and other soft tissues, the altered quality is felt as excessive tension and torsion. Within the bone tissue, it is felt as compression or distortion, while at the joint or suture it is felt as a restricted range. In the fluid system of the body, whether it is the CSF, lymphatic or blood circulation, it is felt as stasis.

A degree of tension is normal and necessary within the soft tissues for the maintenance of structural coherence of the body. When this tension is too much or too little, however, then the structural integrity and body function are affected.

- Too much tension
  Some common indications for this are bony restrictions, reflexes from irritated nerves and internal structures, scar tissue from operations, injuries or muscle spasm. Other reasons are toxic states such as poisoning, anxiety, distress or diseased organs.

- Too little tension
  This is felt mostly in the membranous and ligamentous structures, usually after an injury. Overstretching ligaments, spraining an ankle, for example, weakens the support for the joint. Reduced tone mostly affects the soft tissues that support the internal organs, classically seen in women who have a prolapsed bladder or uterus after multiple births, where support in the pelvic floor becomes weakened.

- Altered feel of tissues due to a chemical imbalance
  This often occurs in swelling (oedema) of inflamed tissues and is the body's response to an allergy, an injury or the inflammatory process of a disease such as rheumatoid arthritis. Various medications such as steroids, epileptic and asthmatic drugs have their own effects on the quality of the tissues.

- Altered feel of tissues due to infections
  Infections are numerous. It might be cystitis, glandular congestion in mumps, tonsilitis or influenza or gastroenteritis – the effects are felt in all the tissues but predominantly in the membranous and fluid aspects of the body. Often a new infection will give a 'boggy' feel to the tissues, whereas a previous severe infection may leave a quality of dryness.

Tissue patterns

So, in summary, the tissues of the body carry a pattern of health and ill health unique to that individual, and the osteopath will be trying to locate what is normal for that person. This is primarily judged by the vitality, amplitude, quality and ease with which the tissues express the motion of primary respiration. The pattern of ill health is a strain pattern so there is poor adaptation of tissues in response to stresses.

Physical injuries or poor postural habits may cause distortion in the tissues, dictated by the direction of the compressive forces or stresses on the body. Such 'stress lines' become ingrained over time, and are felt by the osteopath as torsion, rotation or other patterns of compression/tension within the tissues of the body.

Tissue memory

The body remembers events, both physical and emotional, through its tissues. A classic example is where someone has had a limb removed because of physical injury or gangrene yet still feels the pain in the missing limb. Known as the 'phantom limb' syndrome, the pain is there because of the inscribed neurological and emotional memory.

Tissue memory is a response of the whole body mainly via the nervous system, which pervades all tissues of the body. All the structures of the body, be they bone, muscle, fascia, joint or organs, respond to injury by sending messages to the brain. You may, for example, have a nasty fall, which traps a nerve in the lower back, causing pain down the leg in 'sciatica'. The area of hurt sends messages to the corresponding spinal cord level and the brain areas in charge of that body part. Because the spinal cord records this, pain may linger on long after the nerve has been released. When the injured area has healed, its associated level at the spine may become prone to dysfunction, even after the traumatic event.

Similarly in shingles, a nerve becomes inflamed due to the herpes zoster virus. This causes intense pain that may continue long after the virus has been overcome. The symptoms are worse in individuals that are run down or where the immune system is weak, often with the elderly.

Tissue memory and time

The osteopath ascertains whether the injury is recent or old by the quality of the tissues. As we have seen, a recent injury has the active ingredients of inflammation around it. The tissues reflect this as a swelling, a 'boggy' feel (like a bruised apple) that feels tender on touch. A cold about to start has a similar feel as the body tries to recuperate by mobilizing its lymphatic system and this excessive fluid is felt in the tissues. The freshly established tennis elbow, for example, will appear swollen and tender to touch but the rest of the arm will function well, since a new injury has relatively fewer mechanisms of adaptation.

An old injury means that the body has had time to build up its compensatory mechanisms, one of which is excessive muscular effort. Therefore, the tissues feel fibrotic (like rope) and less fluid. An old illness, such as meningitis, may leave a dehydrated quality in these membranes. An old tennis elbow condition is not that tender to touch, but the bones of the forearm may reveal a twisting pattern of the tissues connecting them and this prevents the bones from functioning fully relative to each other. And in turn, the dysfunctional elbow will affect the movements of the shoulder girdle somewhat.

How the tissues come to be altered – patterning

When there is health, the body is free of any patterns of stress. If all the parts of the body are in a normal relationship, then any stressful events are quickly dealt with. Usually the body can cope with temporary stressful events so it is not adversely affected and with good nutrition and efficient structural mechanics, normal life continues without any great discomfort.

Often, though, areas of the body become conditioned by certain events, such as trauma, long-standing postural and occupational strains, hobbies, falls, illness or emotional stress. These set up patterns of tension and pressure within the tissues to become the body's new pattern of adaptation.

The term 'stress' implies a demand for adaptation to a given situation or 'stressor'. The body responds in its totality, so that all its systems are involved to process and adapt to the challenge. In general, it is only when the body was unsuccessful in returning to its pre-stressed state that it will record and store the 'distress'. This is known as 'potential energy'. It remains held in the body and is experienced as tension. It is well known that being upset or anxious causes tension in the muscles of the neck and shoulders. Over time, this may result in a person having headaches or grinding their teeth during sleep – which does, of course, drain the body's resources.

Stress patterns are inscribed into the tissues by the nervous system and held there by the endocrine system and the psyche. They occur because of the body's ability to adapt immediately to the survival dilemma. In doing so, there are instant advantages for dealing with the situation at hand, but there may be disadvantages in the long run. This is known as 'adaptive behaviour'. However, all adaptive processes require energy to hold that pattern and the long-term effect of this is reduced vitality.

Patterns of 'distress' are recorded as tension/compressive effects on the tissues and certain events have typical presentations. For example, when your car is hit from behind, you may suffer from neck and lower back problems. The pattern in which the tissues are strained is known as a 'whiplash' injury. Other patterns stored in the body may be related to birth trauma, accidents or surgery.

Other types of stress patterns

After an operation or a physical injury that damages the skin and muscles, the body heals by forming scar tissue. Adhesions may also occur in the event of diseased internal organs, such as chronic cystic ovaries. They may also occur following inflammation, immobility or any other condition where there is stagnation and stasis of the motion in the membranes or fluid.

The body forms scar tissue and adhesions by laying down fibres which are not the original elastic tissue. This means that the tissues are held in one place or within a restricted range of motion and after a long period of time this will alter the posture and the comfort of the body. Where there is scarring of tissues supporting the internal organs, their normal sliding and gliding motion within their fascial tissues becomes restricted, which affects their function.

In looking for the cause of discomfort, the entire past and present physiology of the body is considered. All the body structures, together with the interaction of the bones, fluids, membranes and the effects of mechanical dysfunction, play an important part in causing discomfort and ill health.

A typical consultation with an osteopath is illustrated by the case of Mrs Fox, who sought help with headaches.

MRS FOX COMES FOR A CONSULTATION

Mrs Fox walked slowly but deliberately to the chair. She was 52 years old and very pretty, yet her eyes were dull and her face etched in pain. She was suffering from severe right-sided headaches that started over the ear. She needed to be at work and the only way she could get through the day was by taking strong painkillers. This had started only a few months ago, following an operation on her head. Before this, she had suffered badly with dizziness, ringing in the ears and increasing deafness. The operation had successfully removed the culprit – a tumour sitting on the cranial nerve responsible for hearing and balance. All those symptoms had disappeared but now the headaches had taken over in making her miserable.

- Examination using observation and active movements

  Mrs Fox looked pale and her breathing was shallow. Her posture drooped and the head did not feel balanced on the neck and shoulders. As she stood, she held it to the right, snuggled into the shoulder, almost as if she wanted to draw it closer into the body, protecting it.

  There was a slight tendency to wobble, and when she was nudged at the shoulder the gravity line did not correspond to the middle of her body, falling too far forward. However, she managed to walk around without difficulty. While standing, Mrs Fox was instructed to perform some simple movements – bending forwards, backwards, sideways and twisting either way. She found bending the head backwards painful. When asked to stand with her arms outstretched, first with her eyes open and then closed, she managed to maintain her balance in spite of the challenge to her nervous system.

- Sitting examination and palpation

  The skin over the neck and shoulders and in the middle of the back felt clammy and certain areas on the spine were tender to the touch. By cradling the shoulders, gentle movements were introduced into the spinal and rib joints to check for restrictions. By putting one hand on the cranium and the other on the pelvis, the fluid and membranous interconnections were observed.

- Lying examination and specific tests
Because she was suffering with constant headaches, a very simple neurological examination was performed to eliminate any organic pathology within the cranium. The reflexes, muscle power and other tests were found to be within normal limits, as were the blood pressure and pulse. Feeling her abdomen, the area of the liver was slightly tense as was the colon but the glands felt normal.

- While she was lying on her side, I introduced a number of passive motions to the spinal joints. This revealed restrictions in the joints at the top of the neck and upper back. There was also excessive tension in the muscles at the base of the skull and the right side of the neck. The joints of the upper ribs and the pelvis felt limited in their range of movements.

- Examination using primary respiration
When examining the head, I was unable to feel the inherent rhythmic motion properly on the right side, especially at the temporal bone where the ear is. Excessive tension and inertia in the membranes attached to the base of the cranium corresponded to the site of the operation. Testing the bones of the cranium, the right temporal bone refused to budge; its neighbour, the occiput, gave some indication of motion when I engaged a slight compression force into my elbow. This revealed the position of comfort for Mrs Fox's body, and the place where treatment could best be effected.

   The operation to remove the tumour had left scarring in the membranes. As these are attached to the temporal bone they were putting a brake on its motion, causing an asymmetry in relation to the rest of the cranial bones. This was similar to that felt when blowing up a balloon with sellotape on one side. One side blows up nicely, whilst the other side remains stuck. In much the same way, the scarring altered the tissue tension so that it could not permit adequate motion, 'locking up' the cranium and resulting in constant headaches for Mrs Fox. As this was released, the membranes relaxed and the motion of the temporal bone kicked back in on the right side. Gradually the other cranial bones began to articulate with each other. A week later the change had continued to hold, judging by the near symmetry of inherent motion – and indeed Mrs Fox was taking fewer painkillers.

As I have said, the osteopath's tools are observation and palpation. However, she sees and feels not just from the sense organs of the eyes or the hands, but through all her perceptive faculties. This sensing from the whole being comes from previous experience and learning, as well as from the ability to listen and interpret the information from the patient's tissues. Simon illustrates these things rather well.

SIMON'S TROUBLES

Simon was 13 years old and a lot of things were troubling him. He suffered with asthma, had a constant cold, a runny nose and was getting moody. He looked pale but his skin had angry itchy eczema and the bouts of wheezing were increasing.

He was short for his age, underweight and had always been a fussy eater. His mother, Debby, had been unable to breastfeed him and the eczema had started when he was three months old. It had been very severe, but virtually stopped when he was found to be allergic to cow's milk and milk products were eliminated from his diet. It flared up again, however, when he entered his teens. The asthma came on when he was four and unlike the eczema had never gone away. Simon was born without complications, but his first cry was very faint. As an infant, he had been fretful and did not sleep much. This pattern continued, except now he itched during sleep and ground his teeth.

As I watched Simon, it seemed that his rounded shoulders had a permanent home by his ears. His skin was rough and leathery where the last lot of eczema had healed. He looked uncomfortable in his body and in fact, Simon relaxed best when he was fidgeting. On examination, I was aware that his breath was mostly from the upper chest. The muscles at the front of the neck seemed taut. The vertebrae at top of the spine were restricted when he was asked to perform simple movements.

On feeling Simon's tissues, I found tension throughout the body and the tissues felt irritated, dry and hot. The muscles at the base of the skull, the jaw, the shoulders and the left side of the pelvis were very tight and ropey. Feeling for the inherent motions of the body, as one functional unit, was difficult. The overall amplitude felt shallow and lacking in voltage. The head and neck were not in line with the chest and the lower half of the body, feeling almost disjointed. The thoracic diaphragm in particular was tight as were the membranes at the cranial base and behind the breastbone. In the head and face, the base bones were compressed and those forming the sinuses had restricted motion, thereby inhibiting the drainage of mucous membranes. The sacrum and the spinal membranes felt twisted and there were restrictions in the joints of the upper spine, the rib cage and pelvis.

What was the cause of Simon's discomfort?

Young Simon had a lot of complicated physiological factors that led to his discomfort. The strained breathing mechanics showed the difficulty of getting oxygen into Simon's body. The constant sinusitis and a blocked nose did not help. Simon's teeth grinding reflected the tension in his overloaded system and the poor 'fit' between the different bones of the head and face.

Simon's birth took a long time because his head did not have the best match for his mother's pelvis. Although no intervention was needed, the cranial bones could only accommodate the very strong forces generated by the labour through overlapping and becoming distorted. His crying and suckling could not resolve the forces of this birth pattern, which became absorbed into his tissues. This left him not 'fitting properly' into his body, a condition which was reinforced as he grew.

The tension and irritability in Simon's tissues were indicative of an 'over-alert' system, probably from an imbalanced autonomic nervous system – no wonder he was always fidgeting! The powerhouses of this system are influenced by spinal mechanics and the restrictions in Simon's body corresponded to these sites. The resulting tightened blood vessels and laboured breathing meant that poor oxygenation became the 'norm' for Simon.

The motions of primary respiration were laboured throughout the body, which reflected poor vitality in Simon's tissues. The heat within the tissues suggested something of more recent onset, and this may have related to the eczema coinciding with the stress of puberty and a meningitis jab.

Simon's constant runny nose and his eczema were indications of allergy, felt as irritability within the tissues. This was verified by placing possible allergenic factors (in this case, house dust and cow's milk) next to the skin. The response in the inherent motions became disturbed, and the indication was that these substances were currently upsetting the body and were best avoided.

Conclusions drawn from Simon's tissue findings

Several things bothered Simon, the main ones being:

• Poor nutrition and allergies that affected his stature and vitality
• An immune system that functioned disproportionately, becoming over-sensitive and so causing allergies, yet succumbing to infections
• The effect of a vaccination, at puberty, on an imbalanced autonomic nervous system, meant that his body was trying to cope with new stress factors as well as hormones whizzing round

As a baby, Simon was intolerant to cow's milk and eliminating it from his diet had helped enormously. However, the unresolved tensions in the bones and membranes of the cranial base remained, so affecting the cranial mechanics and hence the regulatory and metabolic centres found here. Also, the poor excursion of the rib cage meant that he had never really established good breathing mechanics. Growth requires a lot of energy and Simon's labouring system felt this as an added stress, which reinforced all his problems. Each time there was an energy-consuming process such as growth, vaccinations or emotional upsets, Simon's body became less able to cope, and responded with the bad flare-up of eczema.

How Simon was treated is discussed in the next chapter.

Chapter four

Osteopathic treatment using primary respiration

It is a professional secret, but I'll tell you anyway. We doctors do nothing but aid and encourage the doctor within. All healing is self-healing.

Albert Schweitzer

The power of self-healing

The body has the power to heal and restore us to health. Usually, we have a set life pattern, habitually working too hard, ignoring injuries, not being still enough or eating well, and tiredness is often the body's way of telling us to pause and take stock. But we ignore this and so the body has to shout louder, which it does by giving us pain. Finally, we take note when the problem interferes with our way of life and consciously begin the journey towards healing.

Healing is nature's way of restoring integrity to the injured body tissue, mind or spirit and is ongoing, at the different levels of our being. The healing professions act as aids to this process, but ultimately it is the individual's own body and psyche that does the healing.

Why and how osteopathy promotes self-healing

All types of treatment and medical care rely on the body's innate vitality for healing and optimum recovery. Osteopathy is a hands-on system of medicine that facilitates the body's ability for healing and making its own remedies by removing any hindrances to the inter-relationship of structure and function.

When there is a restriction or distortion in the framework of the body, it alters the space available for its organs and internal structures. As interconnecting fascias and membranous compartments surround the body parts, any tension within these will affect the body's overall comfort and function. The body structure and organs express their function through motion and in order for this to happen freely, they need sufficient room.

The osteopath reads the response of the body to physical or emotional trauma, spiritual neglect, illness and disease as reduced motion in its tissues. By manually restoring movement in the framework of the body and motion in its tissues, the spatial relationships between the body and its organs are improved. This releases the pattern of disturbance in order to allow a new behavioural pattern for the body. The osteopath works on the biomechanical factors, both big and small, so that the body's biochemical and bioelectrical mechanisms are modified. By improving the body's structural integrity and the fluid mechanics of the CSF, the blood supply, venous and lymphatic drainage and autonomic control mechanisms, a better environment is created for bodily functions. As well as treating the area of discomfort, the whole body is encouraged towards a more integrated function, so improving the patient's vitality and reducing the obstacles standing between the patient and health.

Much of the work of the osteopath lies in preventive care as well as giving support in the face of ill health.

Some treatment approaches

The osteopath has many ways of interacting with the body to influence its function, and I will be describing some methods of employing primary respiration during treatment. But it must be emphasized that osteopathy is a philosophy of health and not merely a set of technical procedures which are applied to a given diagnosis. When treating a person with a condition such as asthma, duodenal ulcer or a bad back, the therapeutic methods may appear similar. However, no two people have the same patterns of health and dysfunction, since the body of each reflects their individual lives and different ways of functioning. The method of choice will depend on the person's age, the length of time the condition has been present, how it came about, previous problems, and many other factors. It is the individual's inherent health pattern and the disturbed anatomical and physiological pathways that will dictate the treatment approach.

When the osteopath is working, she is in constant dialogue with the body, 'listening' to the tissues and interacting with them through her input and attention. In turn, the tissues of the patient respond by imparting the locked-up energy from faulty patterns to allow change in their way of functioning. The osteopath feels this as sequences of turbulent activity, stillness and renewed activity until finally there is a transformation into a different tissue pattern, and a corresponding change in motion and function.

Because the same techniques of interaction are used, diagnosis is often combined with treatment. Normally a session begins with the osteopath assessing the strain patterns made up of compression, tension and reduced motion within the tissues. As these begin to change, there is a sense of increased motion, a 'jiggle' in the tissues, followed by stillness when nothing seems to be happening. After a short while, the tissues gently restart their motion. There may be further stillness/activity moments until the tissues have had enough for that session. These phases of motion/stillness/motion can be likened to those of a moving pendulum or a swing. There is motion in the swing (started by the Breath of Life) and therefore a certain amount of kinetic energy. As the swing concludes the arc of motion, there is a moment of stillness before the next arc begins. This momentary stillness holds the potential energy or potency required for the change in direction and speed of the next arc. This moment is valuable, since it holds the potential for change. The point of stillness during treatment is the safest and most powerful place to direct the change and the osteopath works just as much with stillness as she does with motion.

The moment of stillness is related to the motions of primary respiration, which has two phases; between the phases of inhalation and exhalation is a moment of stillness. The osteopath can influence the natural fluctuation of the fluids to bring about the moment of stillness, when energy can be realized and the tissues given an opportunity to change.

While different conditions present with different anatomical, physiological and pathological considerations, some approaches are commonly applied. Most methods of influencing change within the tissues involve restoring the normal relationship of the cranial bones and their membranes, but this will depend upon each person and their underlying physiology. Here are some manoeuvres used by osteopaths working in association with the motions of primary respiration – but of course it is important that they are seen as part of the whole treatment process.

- Push or pull manoeuvres can be used to direct the parts into a balanced spatial alignment with their surrounding structures. The tissues are gently nudged towards the normal position from which they have digressed, as after acute trauma, when misalignments are common.
- The body tissues have the ability to recoil back to a neutral position, just like an elastic band when it is stretched and released. Similarly a strain pattern can be gently exaggerated so that the tissues are taken further into the pattern of fault. Eventually, there is enough build-up of energy or tension to allow a spring back into the correct positional relationship.
- The area at fault is gently separated and allowed to free itself, especially where there is too much tension in the membranes, or there has been a compression or impaction strain of two bones. This is very soothing and also helps to stretch muscles and fascias.
- An injury can traumatize the tissues into working in opposite motions. A blow on the head, for example, can restrict a bone so it does not move in its normal manner, whilst its articulating partner continues its motion in the opposite direction. The body is used to working in a set way, just as we cross one arm or leg over the other habitually. If we instead consciously cross the opposite one, it gives the body a different perspective to work with. Similarly, the membranes attached to the bones can be released by taking the two bones to

their physiological extreme. So one cranial bone is held in the direction it prefers to work in, whilst its neighbour is exaggerated further into the opposite direction, until a balance is achieved and both work together.

• Bones are pliable and plastic, liable to warp under the forces of compression such as during the process of birth, or after an accident. The bone can be remoulded by directly releasing the distortion within it.
• Unwinding the membranes. Membranes of the body can be unwound everywhere, either at one tiny point or in large areas. They can be released specifically for a local problem; for example the membrane that connects the two bones of the forearm or where there is a big mass of membranes, such as the chest or the spine.

Membranes tend to hold tension in torsional patterns, which reflect their position held at the time of a physically or emotionally traumatic event, and also in habitual postures. When this energy potential is released, the membranes unwind in much the same way as the telephone cord. As the receiver dangles, the energy in the length of the cord is released as it unwinds in one direction and then comes to a still point. At this moment, the remaining energy undergoes a transition and spirally unwinds in the opposite direction. So it continues, until all the pent-up energy is dissipated, finally reaching the point of balance when it is without kinks.

One way of unwinding excess tension within the membranes is through repeatedly changing the direction of the tissues. By introducing different directions through internal or external rotation, traction or compression, the tissues are enabled to stop at certain points and alter course. Eventually, the whole process will come to a still point, followed by a final release as the tissues unwind.

Enhancing the treatment

Treatment can be facilitated when the osteopath harnesses the inherent motions of the body, using the breath and the fluctuation of the CSF to work with the two phases of primary respiration.

Asking the patient to hold the breath or allowing a baby to suckle during a treatment helps the membranes to unwind or increase joint mobility, where required. Holding body parts in certain positions, such as pushing the feet down while holding the breath in or out, can also augment the phases of motion of primary respiration and allow the osteopath greater opportunity to balance the tissues.

By using the fluctuation of the CSF, the interchange between the CSF and other fluids of the body and lymphatic functions can be enhanced. These methods are useful when extra nutrition is required, especially where there is a dryness or resistance in the tissues, as is often found in arthritis. They are also useful to clear out congestions, to wash away toxic waste products of the tissues, just like sluicing with a bucket of water.

Since disease manifests itself as a reaction of the whole person to both the internal and external environments, very few complaints can be packaged and labelled as a distinct entity. It is not practical, therefore, to prescribe a set of osteopathic procedures for treating a specific condition, nor does this follow osteopathic philosophy. It is important to remember that osteopathy is concerned primarily with treating the person who is presenting with the ailment, rather than merely addressing the condition. Each session usually lasts between 20 and 30 minutes, where the patient can discuss the behavioural responses of his body in relation to the triggers. For long-term preventive care, he is also supported in introducing changes to his lifestyle so that he can stay healthy.

How often and for how long the patient is seen depends on the acuteness of the condition, and the quality of motion and vitality within the tissues. At the beginning of the treatment programme, a week is usually allowed for the tissues to respond. However, an angry neck, shoulder or other inflamed tissues may be treated within a few days, until they quieten down. Again, where warning signs of a known condition are felt, such as the cough or disturbed breathing patterns of an asthmatic tendency, the patient is seen as often as necessary in order to nip it in the bud. Once the tissues are calmer and the inherent motion within them has improved, then sessions are spaced out over a longer period of time. At the beginning and end of each session, the tissues are assessed for a change in their quality and function. As this improves, treatment can be spaced out over months.

What follows are sections describing some common conditions that affect patients. In most instances, a typical case history is used to illustrate these, along with some explanation as to how such conditions come about, and a treatment approach.

1: Some considerations of ill health

The little things are the big things in the science of osteopathy. . . And it is on those paradoxical gigantic 'little things' that the structure of cranial osteopathy is builded.

Dr William Garner Sutherland

Problems with the workings of the body rarely arise out of the blue. It has usually taken years for that blood pressure to rise or that neck to become arthritic. The duodenal ulcer is probably the end product of prolonged overwork, of a bacterial infection or of not eating balanced meals. But it may have had its origins in mechanical dysfunctions of the spine and distortions within the fascias of the abdomen. Genetics, lifestyle and the effects of previous problems lead to altered physiological mechanisms which, if maintained, often become disease processes.

All doctrines of medicine agree that nutrition and the environment must be right for people to keep healthy. Osteopathy adds that efficient structural and functional relationships of the body play a major role in maintaining wellness. Yet with modern living and all its joys come side effects. Generations have been exposed to pollution, modification of food through refining and processing, and the use of everyday household chemicals. We also experience maintained states of high anxiety. These factors have in large part led to an altered sensitivity of the body's normal physiological mechanisms. And so, we suffer with problems of ill health that were perhaps not so common in our grandparents' time. Allergy is an example of the disruption of the normal ability of the body to function, so that environmental factors overwhelm its defence systems.

As I keep emphasizing, when assessing a patient the osteopath is concerned about the whole person. She therefore considers the normal physiological processes of health within that person, as well as the dysfunctional mechanisms of ill health. Wellness of the body requires maintenance of an appropriate environment for its cells: blood must be reaching every single cell. And, equally, the acidic waste material produced by the tissues must be excreted, so all the drainage mechanisms are just as important. Wellness also requires a balance between body parts and the neural tissues.

The autonomic nervous system (ANS)

The nervous system has an autonomic side, whose main control centre is the hypothalamus in the brain, which regulates the metabolic processes of the body. The autonomic nervous system (ANS) is made up from numerous ganglia found within the cranium, in the muscles of the organs and on either side of the spinal column. There are two divisions: the sympathetic, which is found

Figure 7 THE AUTONOMIC NERVOUS SYSTEM (ANS)

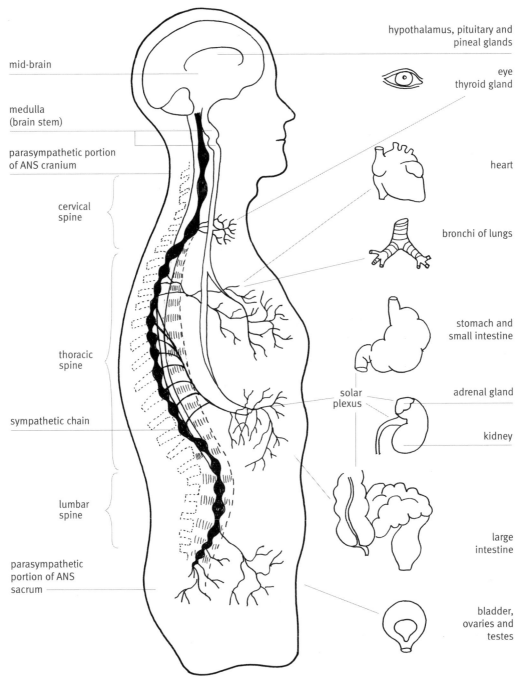

hypothalamus, pituitary and
pineal glands

mid-brain

eye
thyroid gland

medulla
(brain stem)

parasympathetic portion
of ANS cranium

heart

cervical
spine

bronchi of lungs

thoracic
spine

stomach and
small intestine

solar
plexus

adrenal gland

sympathetic chain

kidney

lumbar
spine

large
intestine

parasympathetic
portion of ANS
sacrum

bladder,
ovaries and
testes

primarily at the spinal level; and the parasympathetic, which is at the cranial and sacral levels. These adjust the volume of messages and complement one another so that if the activity of one division increases, the other automatically takes a back seat. The fine-tuning between these divisions helps to maintain a balanced environment within the body.

The ANS has relationships with the internal structures (known as 'viscera'), which stem from the time of embryonic development. To form the different body parts, the embryo divided into segments; the nervous tissue is related to the visceral organs through the spinal segmental pathways (see figure 7). This means that the spine and organs can talk to each other through pathways called reflexes. So the heart, for example, can have a two-way conversation with the spine via the sympathetic nerves at the level of the second thoracic segment, and the gut does the same at the fifth to ninth levels. The 'chatter' is about the regulation of muscle tone and secretion from the glands and organs such as the intestines and their blood vessels. (See the diagram in appendix 1, which shows the inter-relationships of the spinal segments with the different body parts.)

In general, if there is too much activity in the sympathetic division of the ANS, the blood vessels of the organs supplied mainly by the sympathetic system become constricted, so reducing the blood flow. Among other things, this has the effect of inhibiting the circulation within the body, inhibiting the repair mechanism and maintaining anxiety states. When there are poor postural mechanics, the body does not have an efficient relationship with gravity. This creates dysfunctions within the framework, so the overall effect is to increase the sympathetic tone, which in turn will affect the function of the organ supplied at the level of the spinal dysfunction. Equally, when there is irritation of the sympathetic nerve supplying an organ, it talks to its segmental area of origin, lying in the spine as described by the illustration in figure 7, showing the autonomic reflexes between the organs and the framework of the body. As a result, the soft tissues related to this spinal level are less nourished and become ropey, while the overlying skin becomes tender. The osteopath registers these findings, as well as the tension in the surrounding tissues, long before the organ itself sends distress signals. So, when she looks at a spinal segment, she takes into consideration the embryological growth patterns of that segment as well as the mechanical relationship it has with its neighbours. Because of its accessibility, the osteopath can easily work on the spine, cranium and sacrum to influence the functions of the autonomic nervous system and the internal structures it supplies.

HELENA'S DIFFICULTY

Helena was a vibrant, professional lady in her thirties. However, irregular bowel patterns and odd pains had left her feeling below par. She could not remember how or when the change had begun but it was at least two years ago. She tended to be constipated, not having a motion for two days. Sometimes she would have loose stools. Helena's stomach rumbled a lot and she was often bloated, especially after meals and tea. She also had stiffness in the shoulders and middle of the back, but was well otherwise. Of note was an appendectomy in her teens and a car accident in her late twenties. When Helena had investigations of the bowel, they revealed nothing. She was suffering from 'irritable bowel syndrome'. This condition causes a lot of discomfort and tends to affect most people at some stage in life. It is not known to have any organic cause and the episodes are occasionally linked to situations of anxiety, tension and dietetic habits.

When examining Helena I noted that she had a swayback posture. There was a twist in her pelvis and the spinal curves changed where she felt stiff. The muscles attached here, including the diaphragm, were tight, as were the associated vertebral joints. On feeling her abdomen, it appeared that she was tender over the middle and right area and there was tightness over the abdominal fascias. This felt like a downward pulling sensation of the abdominal soft tissues towards the scarring from the appendix operation, which seemed to restrict the natural motion of the bowels and the liver. Normally, because the organs are contained within the flexible fascial coverings, movements of the body cause the organs to be naturally pulled, stretched or compressed. If there is a restriction within these fascias it hinders the position and gliding motion of the internal structures. In Helena, the colon felt as if it were pulled down and sagging, not properly supported by its fascias.

The functions of the gut are regulated by nerve plexuses, which are situated at the spinal level of the waist and the diaphragm. They contain sympathetic pathways and the main one is the coeliac plexus, which lies behind the stomach. It communicates with various abdominal organs and their blood vessels. In this way the gut is the centre point for signals to and from the walls of the chest, diaphragm, liver, stomach, spleen, adrenal glands, kidneys, testes and ovaries. As a result, any problems in the abdominal area or at the respective spinal levels will affect many organs. The plexus has significance because of its instinctive method of communication for feelings such as distrust, fear, elation, sorrow, excitement, anxiety and joy, expressed in apt phrases such as 'gut instinct' or 'centring oneself'. Because it radiates nerves to and from virtually all the abdominal organs and the wall of the chest, the solar plexus orchestrates the effects of emotions and the function of the organs. No wonder Helena could not be specific about where she felt the pain! The sympathetic volume was too high in Helena and so the functional ability of the bowels was affected.

Helena's treatment programme needed to address all these factors. Firstly, her body mechanics needed attention. To begin with, her body was encouraged to function from a position near to its centre or 'midline'. As the cranial and spinal membranes took on a balanced tension the spine became more aligned and the distortions within the diaphragm, abdominal and pelvic fascias were eased. The bowels now had the space and support from their fascias so that natural movements could gradually occur. Then Helena was advised on developing habits so that she did not rush or suppress her motions – or emotions. She was to empty her bowels regularly at the same time each day and to increase her intake of water, vegetables, fruit and fibre, especially at the times when she did not have the runs or felt pain. When she did have pain or diarrhoea, she was to ease off the roughage so that the bowels did not have to work too hard when they felt fragile, but could work on the fibre when they felt stronger. Finally, she joined a yoga and meditation class to help her deal with anxiety situations in the long run.

Sinuses, infections, allergies and intolerances

Facial pain can often be due to sinusitis. Sinuses are air cavities within the bones of the skull. They are made up from two or more bones, and are lined with mucous membranes. Usually as a leftover from a cold, or allergic irritation, the mucous membranes become infected and inflamed and take ages to clear. Sometimes, headaches or a feeling of being muzzy are also due to excessive mucus production and there is often a runny nose or dripping at the back of the throat. The minute movements between the cranial bones help to drain the extra mucus, but when this pumping action is hindered over a period of time, the mucous membranes that line the sinuses become thickened. These unhealthy membranes only know how to produce more mucus. Eating foods such as milk, cheese or chocolate may aggravate the problem since they encourage mucus production. Under the right mix of conditions, this can lead to a vulnerability to upper respiratory tract infections, especially in children. In some cases, such as asthma and glue ear, the immune function can be compromised in two ways. It is not strong enough to fight an infection that usually precedes an episode, and yet it is too sensitive to certain substances as in an allergy.

The body has the ability to resist virtually all types of bacteria, viruses, fungi and parasites, or toxins that might damage its tissues and organs. The natural barriers such as the skin and stomach acid provide resistance to invading pathogens. In the meantime the body's adapting mechanisms make antibodies against bacteria or toxins. But this often takes some time to develop. The cells that protect the body are lymphocytes. These initially develop in the bone marrow and the thymus gland found under the breastbone. They express antibodies and then seed into the lymphoid tissues which are distributed in strategically advantageous areas to intercept the invading organisms before they can spread too widely. These areas are the throat and pharynx, containing tonsils and adenoids, the gut, spleen and bone marrow and lymph glands all over the body connected via the lymphatic channels. However, when there are mechanical problems (as seen in someone who largely breathes through the mouth) the invading bacteria can easily overlook the natural barriers.

The body normally responds to germs by producing antibodies, but in a person who suffers from an allergy, this reaction is too sensitive. Substances that are harmless to most people are read as enemies and the body makes antibodies against these. Although allergy is a state of hypersensitivity of the person as a whole, it manifests in a particular area of the body. Asthma affects the lungs, while hay fever affects the eyes and sinuses; other forms are eczema and hives and all of these are reactions to substances that we breathe, touch, eat or drink. Some natural allergens include cow's milk, nuts, wheat, pollen and dust. Working long hours can deplete the body's resources too, making the immune system more vulnerable. These can be controlled somewhat with changes to diet and lifestyle. Where there are synthetic allergens such as insecticides, fertilizers, colourings, sweeteners or detergents, the immediate environment needs to be addressed. Because the body remembers its last encounter with an allergen, it sets up a system for making the antibodies quickly for the next episode. As a result, chemicals such as histamine are released to give the immediate reaction of allergy, with symptoms of a rash, itching, wheezing, runny nose or eyes, hives, bronchial spasm, headaches or vomiting. These symptoms may either occur immediately or be delayed for up to 72 hours.

Intolerance or sensitivity are subtle variations when the immune system over-reacts. But this reaction occurs slowly and the symptoms are not so obvious, taking months or even years to develop, and do not necessarily include the body's release of histamine. Often an ingredient in food causes irritation, such as gluten in cereals, caffeine in coffee, sugar, or cola drinks. This may be due to a lack of physical ability to cope with the food substance. Shortage of the lactase enzyme, for example, results in intolerance to dairy products. In some cases the body's defences become so over-reactive that they attack molecules in certain parts of the body, such as the gut. Eating foods that can inflame the bowels, combined with exposure to bugs, antibiotics, medication, anxiety or an overgrowth of the yeast organism cause the bowel to become 'leaky'. As a result the bowel absorbs large, undigested molecules, which the body mistakes for an invader and so the digestive tract produces symptoms of an allergy. Consequently, the tone of the stomach and intestines is lowered, leading to a longer emptying time. The symptoms of constipation and poor digestion, similar to those suffered by Helena, may be due to the reduced motility of the gut.

There are many different ways in which intolerances can present. Children with a sensitivity to food additives may become hyperactive or fatigued. This is often accompanied by changes in concentration, memory, moods, thinking and behaviour or anxiety. Often in the presence of an allergy there is an underlying factor that may have caused hypersensitivity. It is not unusual for a person to be sensitive to one substance now and to different substances in years to come and this may be partly attributed to long-term effects of unresolved stress on the body. This often leads to a compromised immune function where the effects of allergy and intolerance are compounded – as we saw earlier (pages 59–60) in the many problems of Simon.

SIMON'S TROUBLES

Simon was a sensitive person and his physical problems were reactions of hypersensitivity and a compromised immune function. His main difficulties were eczema, asthma and allergy to milk, with intolerances to dust and other food substances.

His osteopathic care required attention to all of him – his physical, emotional and spiritual needs. His treatment programme required total structural integration, from head to feet. This meant integration of the chest with the rest of the body, improving the immune function and retuning the autonomic nervous system. This was addressed by rebalancing the area of sympathetic outflow at the neck, dorsal spine, ribs and associated soft tissues, whilst the parasympathetic partner was attended to from the cranium and pelvis. In order to help with the immune function, the lymph flow was addressed through using fluctuation of the CSF, improving the mechanics of the chest, its membranes and fascia. Lymphatic function is sensitive to alterations in the biomechanics of the chest and abdomen – so the restrictions in the soft tissue and fascial continuity in the neck, chest and the coverings of the chest and abdominal structures were also released.

Simon had also had a difficult birth: helping his body to release the retained strains meant that his body could work with greater efficiency. However, because the tissues were fatigued, he was treated very specifically per session and his body was given time to reorganize itself and adapt to each treatment. Gradually, as the diaphragm became less tense the ribs became more mobile and moved easily with each breath, the passage of the lymph through the chest began to improve and this helped him to fight off infections.

Over a period of months and keeping to a strict diet, the physiological responses of Simon's body, although still reactive, were not so angry. He was becoming a calmer person, more focused and coping better with situations that used to get him worked up. As the areas showing allergic reactions – nasal and facial bones – were helped to regain their motion, gradually the cells of the unhealthy mucous membranes were replaced by healthy ones, which only produced mucus when required to do so. Occasional blips in his diet and upsetting situations meant he still had his ups and downs but on the whole he was much more comfortable.

2: Physical trauma – accidents and injuries

The mechanical cause of disease is more deeply rooted and of greater fundamental significance than the chemical.

Harold Ives Magoun

Accidents and injuries are an inevitable part of life. The body has a remarkable capacity to accommodate and recover from falls, car accidents and so on. In response to these events the body adapts by changing its behaviour patterns so that although we may suffer the odd bruise and ache we do not give the event a second thought. These compensatory mechanisms, however, can be high maintenance and use up a lot of available energy. And, over a period of time, they lead to further effects so that the original cause becomes a relatively insignificant aspect of the eventual outcome. Under certain circumstances the body becomes overwhelmed, so that the compensatory mechanisms break down. This is accompanied by the appearance of symptoms that are apparently unrelated to the original event, sometimes even years later.

Whiplash injury

One of the commonest types of injury is 'whiplash', often associated with car accidents. This occurs when there is a rapid and abrupt change in direction as a result of an impacting force from behind. There is a momentary loss of control of the head and neck. The effect on the tissues is much like the cracking of a whip and this type of injury usually traumatizes the soft tissues of the neck. Because the body is a unit, however, all its parts are disturbed, and the response from the tissues is manifold. There is a profound physiological and psychological shock to the whole body. The violent assault usually occurs unexpectedly, so there is no time or awareness to prepare oneself and it is difficult to understand what has happened. Sometimes symptoms appear straightaway or in a matter of hours. Usually, however, there is a delay and the body responds in days, weeks or even months after the trauma.

SUNITA'S ACCIDENT
When Sunita came into the consulting room she looked fragile, vulnerable and much older than her 35 years. She supported her head in her hands because it felt too heavy. She was suffering primarily from intense pain and stiffness in the neck, but virtually all her body was one big hurt. She felt bruised, nauseous, had an upset stomach and felt dizzy. Her eyes were sore and it was difficult to focus. Her chest ached and she had not been able to sleep since the accident, prior to which she had enjoyed good health.

Waiting at the traffic lights, Sunita had glanced in the rear-view mirror and read the disastrous scene before it happened. A driver in a laden pick-up van came into her at speed, using her vehicle for a braking device and shunting it forwards. Sunita had felt the full impact. She hit her head on the headrest and, although not concussed, immediately developed a headache and pins and needles in the arms. Investigations at the local hospital thankfully revealed no breaks and she was sent home with a neck-collar and tablets for pain and inflammation.

Upon examination, Sunita's body felt to me as if it were still in a state of shock. Her tissues felt as if they were repeating the strain pattern of being hit from behind. Her body seemed to be functioning from a place yards in front of her, almost where her body would have been, had she not been strapped in the car. Sunita's neck was very tender to touch and the surrounding membranes and soft tissues were angry. The vertebrae in the middle of the neck felt strained and unstable, but the area between the shoulders felt rigid. As Sunita had hit her head on the headrest, this locked up the base of the skull, which felt very compressed. This compression was also felt through the top of the neck and upper back. When I assessed the tension in the cranial and spinal membranes, they felt very taut and irritable, almost 'whipped up'. The nervous system felt charged and the spinal highway was extremely busy, causing the autonomics to the inner organs, especially the gut, to be unsettled. Sunita also had blurred vision. Since the muscles of the eyes receive their autonomic supply from nerve ganglia at the neck and the upper back, their function had also been affected. The whole spine together with the sacrum felt as if it had been shot upwards and then slammed back down, jamming it within the pelvis. In the meantime, the tissues of the lungs and chest felt as if she had taken a huge breath in and had difficulty in breathing out again. When she saw the van coming, she had probably braced herself and held her breath. Although the seat belt had stopped her from being thrust through the windscreen, it had strained the rib joints at the front of the chest, so breathing deeply or sneezing was painful.

Because of her difficulty in lying down, Sunita was treated sitting. Although her physical body had been restrained by the seat belt, the force of the hit was still continuing, taking her 'midline' with it. This made Sunita appear to be disconnected within herself and also with the world; she said afterwards, 'I feel like I am all over the place . . . not like me.' Initially the treatment was to help her re-establish her equilibrium, in order to release the shock and calm down the neural tissues. To help her body release the forces of the trauma, the membranes were gently unwound until they felt more balanced. This was enough to make her comfortable. Three days later, Sunita no longer suffered from the dizzy spells and was sleeping better. Although she was still in pain, her tissues were cranking into action again.

Gradually, as I released the compressive effects from the fascias and balanced the spinal ligaments, there was better alignment of the spine. Once the motions at the sacrum and bones of the cranial base were restored, the strain at the top of the neck and the head eased. Balancing the soft tissues attached to the cranial base bones, shoulder girdles, diaphragm and the pelvic floor enforced the interconnectedness of the body. Releasing the chest and rib restrictions helped to ease the forces from the seat belt so that Sunita could breathe freely. The aching in the upper back soon improved and gradually, over a period of months, the head and neck became more stable. Sunita's confidence returned and she felt stronger emotionally and physically. She was fortunate to have been referred quickly, so the effects of the trauma had not had time to set in and create secondary effects.

Storage of physical stress and its effects

JOE'S FOOT
Joe had crushed his heel in a car accident. Somehow, during the accident, Joe had slammed his heel on to the brake and the force of the impact had crushed it. He had not sustained any other breaks or injuries. Twenty years later, he came to the clinic with knee pain. The following is an account of what was going on in Joe's body.

The body is basically a collection of cells which are bathed in moving fluids, giving it a biodynamic structure that works under the normal compressive forces of gravity. When there is a physical trauma, the body reads this as added compression forces from the impact and the direction from which that impact is coming: the osteopath will feel this as compression and tension within the tissues, held in the direction of the hitting force. As the body absorbs the energy of the collision or injury, its fluid function becomes modified so that these additional forces can work with the existing physiology. How strongly the injury becomes ingrained depends on the degree of the neurological imprint on to the tissues and this is related to the intensity and duration of the injury. A severe injury will send substantial messages to the brain, with millions of signals from the damaged tissues screaming up the spinal cord into the brain. Excessive firing of impulses within the brain and spinal cord therefore record a heavy imprint, which may relay memory messages long after the injured area has healed. Where there been a damaging trauma that was accompanied by severe pain or emotional upset, the brain's emotional centres relay the hurt into the body tissues, so adding to the imprint of the trauma. When Joe crushed his foot, the hypothalamus also recorded shock and fear and this too was relayed into his tissues, increasing their tension. The effects of any previous accidents or illnesses will influence the body's ability to recover from these combined forces.

The force of a physical trauma represents substantial kinetic energy being absorbed into the body. Some of this added force or energy into the body is dissipated, through movement (such as falling). The healing force of the body immediately responds by releasing some force as heat (as in inflammation, or fever), while the remaining energy, related to the directional forces of the impact, is stored in the tissues as potential energy. The response of the body is to take care of its immediate survival needs with the intention of resolving the stored energy later. For example, while Joe's foot is in the recuperative phase, his body improvises its structure so that he can carry on functioning as near normally as possible. It does this by enclosing the energy from the direction factor. After a week or two, as Joe's body works around it, this potential energy becomes integrated into the tissues. There, it may stay unresolved for years after the initial trauma, in the forgotten background, until such a time as the system becomes overloaded because of some new event.

And indeed, when I examined Joe I was aware of an enclosed area of compression felt through the tissues of the heel bone (calcaneum). This followed what felt like a line of force directed upwards through the axis of the leg, which had displaced the alignment of the axis or the tibia with the femur, so straining the knee.

Unresolved trauma

Often, the effects of trauma remain hidden because there is no obvious fracture or concussion, as we saw in the case of four-year-old Lucy who lost her speech (pages 34–35). If it is not complicated a fracture is often left to heal by itself, usually immobilized in plaster. The more severe breaks are often put together by screws, plates or pins and then immobilized. Occasionally, a broken bone will fail to set properly and if left alone may heal with deformity, especially in the elderly. Although the broken bone naturally heals, the direction and force of the trauma also need to be resolved so that the relationship of the body parts can accommodate the break efficiently. The body's capacity to heal bone can be helped by encouraging the motions of primary respiration within the bone tissues so they 'breathe' properly. Rebalancing the axis of the affected limb and the adjacent body parts, taking the unnecessary tension out of the attached membranes and coaxing the trauma out of the tissues, offers the body the best possible chance of recovery.

Physical trauma that is unresolved within the body tissues is a significant contributing factor towards ill health. The normal physiology and current state of health play a great part in how the body is affected by trauma. A woman is less stocky than a man and therefore absorbs a greater degree of stress from a similar impact. Existing health problems at the time mean that the body is already under some sort of strain. How the body is affected by a trauma also depends on the direction of its forces at the time of trauma. One of the worst cases I have seen was Sarah, who at the time when her car was hit from behind was talking on the mobile phone and twisting to look at her husband. The combination of the twisting vectors added to the forces of being hit from behind was so great that it escalated pre-existing problems. Sarah's body was already burdened from having had a hysterectomy and two back operations. She was born with a defect that causes a spinal vertebra to slip forwards in relation to the one below it. This instability had required operations to fuse the vertebrae, many years prior to the accident. The impact of the hit, however, had destabilized the entire spinal mechanics. As a result, Sarah's health declined, the membranes and connecting fascias remaining traumatized so that the blood, nerve and lymph channels became disturbed. This affected the function of her organs as the fluid interchanges became impaired and she started to suffer from an irritable bowel. Because of the impaired body mechanics and the mental pain she experienced, eventually the hormonal and enzyme mechanisms became so altered that the thyroid function was affected.

When Sarah came for treatment, two years after the event, she arrived with pain in her neck and shoulders. In addition, stasis within the tight fascias and membranes had led to deteriorating general health. Because the tissues prior to the accident were already physiologically disadvantaged, the trauma of the accident had far-reaching effects on the whole body. Sarah became edgy and fatigued easily. The total body mechanics and its fluid function were addressed, and gradually Sarah felt less pain. But although she was now more comfortable, she was still anxious; her story is followed in the section on life changes, on pages 128–9.

The effects of minor trauma such as trips and falls are especially important in the growing child. As Keri, a toddler, learns to walk, she inevitably lands square on the bottom, jamming the sacrum between the pelvic bones. Usually this has no undue consequences and because of her resilience, she picks herself up and is off again. However, as Still said 'cause and effect are perpetual' so that the fall (cause) results in the pelvic mechanics being less efficient; the effects of this may not show up until much later. As a child, Keri falls on her bottom in the playground. She cries, but a kiss and a cuddle make it all better and a few days later the incident is forgotten. But because there is already reduced motion within the sacrum and membranes, the way the spine develops is affected. The results are a predisposition to later problems – such as a weakness of the back or menstrual irregularities. Repeated spinal compression can also affect the balance of the autonomic nerves emerging from the spine as they supply the insides. The effects on the internal organs may be a predisposition to an irritable bowel, bedwetting, poor breathing or a multitude of related problems.

All children have knocks and injuries and not all of these need attention since the body is resilient and can usually cope. However, the nature of the event and the emotional dynamics of the trauma are important factors in how the body deals with the trauma. If there are any jolts to the spine, especially at its base, or knocks to the head, the body will absorb these forces. The behaviour of the child in response to such minor trauma is the key to judging the effects on the whole body system: if the child's normal behaviour alters, and he becomes restless, aggressive or too quiet, then a second opinion should be sought. The child's development may continue to be affected by these forces, which need to be to be resolved so that the body does not continue to bear additional stresses.

The effects of the forces of physical trauma and the adaptation of the body around them are continual. As a result, each new added force brings with it a new pattern of adaptation so that the body mechanics are constantly changing to find positions of comfort. But they may do so at the cost of compromising nerve function, blood flow and other physiological processes, using up the body's energy reserves. Because osteopathy works with the inter-relationships between environmental forces, structure and function in terms of motion and movement, it is highly successful in the treatment of the effects of physical trauma, accidents and injuries.

3: Stress and distress

ROSIE'S DISTRESS

Rosie was 37 years old, overweight and irritable. Her neck was painful and she only wanted a 'quick fix' so she could return to work. She did not report much in her history, except for the odd cold and back pain. Upon examining her, I felt there was indeed a problem – the neck vertebrae were 'locked' and associated with this was tightness in the muscles around the spine as far as the waist. The bones at the base of the cranium felt compressed, whilst the membranes attached to them, especially at the back part of the head near the area of the brain stem, felt as if they were dragging. The fascias covering the throat, middle back over the kidneys and adrenal glands held an abnormal level of tension. These areas coincided with hormonal glands, and in terms of metabolism and probably hormonal function, this body had seen better days.

Rosie was given first-aid treatment through manipulation of the joints and easing of the soft tissues. At the end of the session, she was advised that in view of the findings, she needed regular sessions. Rosie's body was sluggish, lacking in vitality and yet there was a lot of potential for improvement. She agreed that she wanted to sort herself out in the long term. She also revealed that she had a poor relationship with her father who was sick, and this grieved her.

After a few treatments, she reported that she had no idea why but she was much better. She could not explain what had happened, but said she felt more able to cope, had begun walking regularly and decided she wanted to come off anti-depressants. Rosie had not revealed this initially, but she had a history of mild depression. Helping the bones of the cranial base and sacrum to open had allowed the cranial membranes to lift. This in turn had eased the sagging effect on the brain stem and the overall hormonal balance. Now, a year later, she pops in for an occasional 'top up'. Although she is still overweight, she is much happier, full of energy and zest for life. She rarely has a cold; she feels she has become more tolerant and is now able to enjoy being with her father.

Rosie had felt that there was not much wrong with her beyond the stiff and painful neck. Her tissues, on the other hand, revealed her response to a stressful scenario and needed help to counter this. Her problems related in part to the painful unresolved situation with her father and in part to deteriorating spinal mechanics. Integrating the structure and function of the body had helped her to deal better with normal life although she could not pinpoint how.

Most osteopaths believe that the treatment they give extends beyond the physical and can help the person deal with emotions and the psyche. Through the sensitivity of her touch, the osteopath appreciates that, yes this patient has a bad back, but he is also angry. Equally, a child's sleeping pattern may be disturbed by a fall, or the death of a grandparent. In cases of severe injury or upset a patient may feel a sense of 'psychic dislocation', a feeling of the whole body being out of itself, or sometimes a limb or part of the body being disowned. In the process of treatment usually both the patient and the osteopath may feel this dissipate as the body comes into balance. Even though the patient may not be able to explain this inner change, he can certainly sense that some shift has occurred.

Stress is defined in Dorland's medical dictionary as 'the sum of the biological reactions to any adverse stimulus, physical, mental or emotional, internal or external, that tends to disturb the organism's homeostasis; should these compensating reactions be inadequate or inappropriate, they may lead to disorders.' The adverse stimulus is known as the stressor and it causes the body systems to alter their normal homeostatic balance in a state known as 'allostasis'. This change sets up a state of compensated body function to help us to deal with the stressor. Once the stimulus is over, the normal homeostatic balance is restored. So when the body meets a bug, which is the stressor, the normal balance of the body shifts in order to resist infection. The regulatory mechanisms up the thermostat so that extra heat, which we feel as a fever, kills off the offending microbe, after which a normal temperature resumes.

Ordinarily, we tend to work better when there is a subliminal level of anxiety or 'pressure'. A new project or challenge, for example, gives us the drive to renew performance and is essential for survival and responding to the daily challenges of life. We have a sensitive stress response for this very purpose. But too many challenges mean that stress is not beneficial but damaging. In medical terms, stress means that a group of chemicals, mainly cortisol, adrenaline and noradrenaline, are released into the body. They are produced whenever the body experiences an excessive load, whether it is too much exercise, mental pressure, toxicity, allergenic substances or an accident. These stress conditions might be physical (such as stubbing the toe) or chemical (such as poor diet or lack of oxygen) or emotional (such as excitement, fear or anger), but the response is through the entire body. Grief, shock or other emotions or high-pressure work are not just expressed in the mind, but are borne by the body as well. When the demands become too much they create an overload: the ability to cope is exceeded and this is known as 'distress'. All types of stressors produce a similar set of responses in the physiology and psychology of the body, known as the general adaptive response. The mechanism for orchestrating this is through the complex neural, hormonal and immune pathways.

The stress response

Certain chemicals, the product of many cells in the nervous, hormonal (endocrine) and defence systems of the body, are released in baseline rhythms to maintain a balanced internal body environment. This 'neural-endocrine network' has a profound effect on our physiology and psychology. When stress is experienced the body mechanisms quickly release the appropriate chemicals and hormones, but in greater quantities than usual. This creates an internal imbalance, which is temporarily needed to protect the body. As a result, several responses occur. The higher centres of the brain, the cerebral cortex (the outer layer of the brain), the limbic system (the part of our brain that governs our most basic emotions) and the hypothalamus (under the cortex) bring about behavioural adaptations so that we become vigilant, alert and cautious. For example, pain coming from the foot will first be translated in the hypothalamus into an emotion such as fear, and within milliseconds a thought from the cerebral cortex will occur: 'my foot is broken', followed by another thought: 'I must not take any weight on it'.

What goes on in the brain has a direct effect on the body. Messages circulate all over the body to stimulate the release of the chemicals needed to counter stress. So, although the sensations that we experience and name as stress, such as anxiety or even excitement, start in the hypothalamus, the actual physical response is modulated in the body, by the autonomic component of the nervous system. The 'thermostat' for this is set in the hypothalamus, which regulates the metabolic processes by releasing substances into the bloodstream. This system maintains balance through its two divisions (see pages 67–69 for more on the autonomic nervous system or ANS). The sympathetic branch of the ANS is found primarily at the spinal level and generally regulates arousal, so that the heart beats faster, blood pressure rises and sweating increases. The parasympathetic branch, on the other hand, is found at the cranial and sacral levels and it induces relaxation. In response to stress, large parts of the sympathetic branch may discharge at the same time. The body can therefore perform vigorous muscle activity, responding far beyond the normal expectations. The main agents responsible are cortisol and adrenaline released from the adrenal glands, at the top of the kidneys. As a result, the production of glucose is increased so that the body can mobilize its energy stores for escape, while both wound repair and body functions that are not vital for escaping from a stressful situation are suppressed.

We are well suited to dealing with short-term physical emergencies; the physiological stress response provides us with phenomenal bursts of energy, sometimes enabling us to perform near-miraculous feats. The body does this by prioritizing its functions so there is plenty of immediately available energy to deal with the problem. So, when faced with a mugger you decide to run. Glucose and nutrients are then instantly mobilized from the liver, fat cells and muscles to feed the area of the body that is in hyper-drive. In order to get the glucose and oxygen to the legs as quickly as possible, the heart rate and breathing increases, as does the blood pressure. During this time of acute stress it makes sense to hold off time- and energy-consuming projects until the emergency is over. Digesting dinner is a slow process and anyway there is not enough time to derive the benefits. It may be advantageous to have longer legs while running for your life, but now is not the time to be growing them – and so growth processes are inhibited. Dealing with bugs breathed in or spotting aberrant cells in the body will have to wait until later. While escaping, reproduction is not practical and therefore desire is inhibited, as is ovulation and the production of testosterone. You trip and break your wrist, but thanks to the stress response going into shock is delayed. Natural analgesics are released so that you do not feel the pain and get up straightaway to carry on sprinting. As your senses have become heightened you can hear and see more acutely; suddenly, you remember a short cut through the alleyway, thanks to the improved memory and sharpened sensory and cognitive areas of the brain, and you escape. After a while, the sweat dries, breathing and heart rate return to normal, the wrist hurts and you badly want a doughnut with a cup of tea!

The responses of the body to such a scenario are, fortunately, not required regularly. Stress has become a popular term that refers to demands imposed on us from a large array of circumstances. Through its immediate reflexes the whole body is put 'on alert', and creates the excessive energy needed to react quickly. But modern living entails responding to situations where this immediate physical response is often inappropriate. Our everyday life is filled with worrying about finding a parking space, traffic jams, meeting deadlines, promotion, paying bills, relationships. We have little time, into which we squeeze far too much. Such states of anticipation activate the same physiological processes evolved for responding to acute physical emergencies, such as running for your life. These psychological and social stressors can be turned on for months at a time so that we remain in a prolonged state of altered balance. For example, you might be worried about meeting your daughter's college fees, your partner's medical results and you are late for a meeting with the boss who is being a pain. So when you see your car getting a parking ticket, the body has an immediate rush in preparing for the instant action. The stress neuro-hormones are already in the bloodstream because of all the other things you are worried about. You can't lynch the traffic warden; if you argue it might disperse some of the newly produced stress hormones, but you will probably still be angry and frustrated – those chemicals are lurking in the body, filling up the stress level file. The excessive energy created by an event like this needs to be dispersed immediately, but when this does not happen the body remains 'on alert' to some degree. Being in a hyper-alert state can in the long run lead to fatigue, lethargy and compromised responses to infections or accidents, no matter how mild.

An emotional shock, physical trauma or an ongoing situation such as doing a job you hate all result in the release of the same stress neuro-hormones. Sometimes, the source of stress does not go away and becomes a part of everyday experience, such as working with someone you dislike. The body then continues its adaptive responses to the point where they become detrimental to health. Surprisingly, we may suffer from odd symptoms even when life is treating us well. If there has been a period of stress or a stressful event in the past the effects may still continue, perhaps in symptoms such as the headache that comes on at the weekend, or an illness on holiday, when it seems that the body has time to fall ill.

The prolonged physiological effects of stress are many and variable, affecting both psychological and physiological processes. For example, increased blood cortisol is characteristic of high stress levels, but it is also a common feature in people diagnosed with melancholic depression. This disease is characterized by such disturbances in personality as increased anxiety, vigilance, obsessive behaviour, hyperarousal, aggression and feelings of worthlessness. These are similar symptoms to those of someone who has been under prolonged stress. One of the body's responses here is to modify the metabolism of food. The liver can make glucose for extra heat and energy, whilst the mineral salts present in sweat are modified to regulate the blood and fluid volume of the body. If this continues over a long period of time it can lead to:

• High blood sugar levels, which may eventually lead to diabetes mellitus
• Poor development of cartilage, which may give aching in the joints
• Reduced absorption of calcium from the intestines, which may
  lead to osteoporosis
• Reduced inflammatory responses, so that injuries take longer to heal
• Increased susceptibility to allergy and intolerance to substances
• Water retention

How stress and infectious stimuli affect the body's defences against diseases is not yet completely understood. In this era, we generally tend to suffer with slow, chronic ailments such as asthma, cardiovascular disease, cancer, irritable bowel syndrome, premenstrual tension, migraines, chronic fatigue syndrome or allergies, and stress appears to play a large part in contributing to these conditions. Where stressors are long-term it seems that the endocrine and autonomic nervous systems continue to modulate the immune system so that its function is undermined. There is a communication network between the nervous, hormonal and immune systems that assures the constancy and integrity of body cells and tissues. The hormones from the pituitary, adrenal, thyroid, thymus and pancreas – growth hormones, oestrogen and testosterone – all interact with the neural and immune systems. The brain modulates activity of the immune system in part, via the hypothalamus; through its connection with the emotional centres in the limbic system, the hypothalamus relates to feelings of joy, happiness, mental pain, grief, anxiety and depression. A person who has been under stress therefore also may experience mood changes, irritation, poor concentration, tiredness and inability to sleep. This is often followed by lack of vitality, feeling worn out and a compromised ability to fight off infections. Eventually, we may suffer the long-term effects of poor digestion, reduced libido and fertility, and, in children, growth problems.

Storage of stress and emotion

The mechanisms of stress can often be triggered when we cannot release or come to terms with emotions. Although we might think that we have no inner conflict, the body holds the unresolved situation in storage. Emotions such as grief, fear, anger and resentment or hurt are stored as a tissue pattern, causing the tissues and membranes to 'freeze up' so that little motion is felt within them. Feelings of pain, shock and resentment may be linked to a physical event such as an accident or a medical procedure. These enduring tissue patterns represent the mind/body interface, since the tension ingrained in the membranes around the physical event is of a behavioural/psychological nature. Sometimes a memory of the long-forgotten event may surface when the patterns are released. Often it may not, but there is a sensation of 'lightness' in the body.

People often complain of tension and stiffness in the neck and shoulders when they are under pressure. Certain areas appear to be more susceptible to housing stress; these include the neck, the head, the chest, solar plexus and lower back. There is a sense of compression or 'locking' within these tissues, especially the membranes covering the heart and lungs, the diaphragm and the intestines. In addition, the autonomic nervous system feels out of sync, something which can be identified in the quality of the body tissues: the skin may feel itchy over certain areas, particularly the spine, and it may be tight, clammy or hot. Where there has been a physical injury, the area expresses the inherent motions poorly, as it 'houses' the emotional trauma linked to the event. This area then becomes a fixed point around which the body can adapt to compensate for the hurt.

As we have seen, one of the first responses to stress is the activation of the hypothalamus, occurring through its connections with the spinal cord and limbic forebrain via the fluid compartments of the brain. This concept is useful for the osteopath, who can use the cerebrospinal fluid circulation to influence the immune function and encourage the body to release its patterns of stress and emotions. Moreover, the parasympathetic division of the ANS is housed primarily at the cranial base and at the sacral spinal cord, while the sympathetic division is found along the spine. The osteopath can easily make use of these parts to access and influence the ANS functions.

JOHN'S CHRONIC FATIGUE

John had been suffering from chronic fatigue, was prone to infections that took ages to shift, and was generally feeling 'out of sorts'. His digestion was fine, although he had occasionally felt bloated. He had been suffering like this over the last two years, following an episode of influenza. All blood tests and investigations from the GP revealed nothing abnormal. John had been on several courses of antibiotics but the colds still kept coming every three to four weeks. His condition made him feel rather low; he was unable to exercise and although he had a successful job as a banker, he felt unfulfilled. John was 45 years old and happily married with two lovely teenage daughters.

John believed that all he needed to get better was to strengthen his immune system. I asked him about his life story, and it emerged that the original symptoms coincided with the death of his favourite sister from cancer. Further digging revealed that he had had a mentally and physically disabled brother who had died many years ago. John's mother was an alcoholic and his father had relied heavily upon him in looking after both the mother and brother. Mentally and emotionally he had to support his mother through her drinking, whilst physically he had to carry his brother around and deal with his needs.

John had not consciously registered the emotional turmoil of his earlier years and regarded his childhood as normal, 'no big deal'. His body, however, had a different story to tell. It had recorded that the survival of this young man would be at a price – that of the immune function.

As I examined John, the overall quality of his tissues felt weary, and vitality was lacking. John's eyes were lack-lustre and there was a general greyness over his face. He had a slumped posture with rounded shoulders and the long muscles of the back and neck felt ropey and sagging. The breath was shallow and the diaphragm felt as though it were held in a vice, so that poor movement of the rib cage and lungs had compromised the drainage of the lymphatic channels. At the stomach level, there was again a feeling of tension over the solar plexus and liver areas.

John's childhood had been extremely stressful but his body had adapted very well over the years to help him cope. Over a period of time, beginning in his childhood, the thermostat set to counter stress was raised and now elevated levels of stress neuro-hormones had become a normal state of affairs. The adaptive response had compensated so much that even though John now had few stressors in his life, the long-term effect was a compromised immune function. The body's defence mechanisms took a big knock in trying to fight off the initial episode of influenza; the immune system was laid low. John's body just could not pick up, and he was diagnosed with 'chronic fatigue syndrome'. Although he was now surrounded by a loving family and in a successful job, his body needed help in retuning the thermostat just enough to allow the body to say 'I don't need the effects of all those stress chemicals now, that part of my life is over and I've moved on.'

John's treatment, over several months, involved using his framework to release the effects of tension that had become an integral part of him. The cranial base was released and this, together with work balancing the sacral base and fluid fluctuations in the body, helped to fine-tune the neuro-endocrine-immune interactions. Treatment to the spine, together with unwinding the membranous tension between the head and shoulder girdles and the thorax and pelvis, helped to support the lymphatic system and immune function. The breathing was helped by getting the diaphragm to relax and the joints of the rib cage to function without any restrictions. The autonomic setting of his stomach and intestines were balanced by working on the spinal levels and the solar plexus, which helped with digestion.

The final recovery for John came when the three aims of treatment were achieved. These were the integration of the autonomic-endocrine-immune function; easing out the compression held in the emotional areas of the body; and reconnecting with memories of a childhood laden with huge responsibilities. This work enabled John to relate his childhood experiences in a different light, and allowed his body to create a shift in the way it responded to stress. John's health and energy levels returned and after six months he hadn't had a cold or sore throat. He also regained enough confidence to consider changing his occupation. With encouragement he followed his childhood dream, and became a full-time artist. Now, when infections do take hold the immune system wins the battle and recovery is generally swift.

Distress is a major factor in our becoming unwell. The body tries to adapt and compensate, but eventually imbalance in all its systems means that its functions become altered. In some people this may lead to depression (as with Rosie) or to anxiety attacks. Certain people are especially vulnerable, particularly if there is an underlying psychological or psychiatric problem, when appropriate help is essential. Although working on the physical body to restore balance brings enormous relief, it is important to check how we can alter our response to distress. Osteopathy can greatly lower the tension patterns for someone who is experiencing high anxiety or has residues of unexpressed emotions that are preventing the body from functioning to its full capacity. Equally, learning and understanding about ourselves, our coping mechanisms and lifestyle are important steps towards total healing and to enjoying a better way of being.

4: Dental difficulties and jaw problems

MICHAEL'S BITE

Twelve-year-old Michael had mysteriously started to suffer from seizures. Although brain investigations revealed nothing abnormal, the seizures took on an atypical epileptic form. He was on medication, but his studies were suffering. Michael was wearing braces, and it emerged that prior to the onset of the seizures he had received orthodontic treatment to restructure his bite.

On examination, I found there was poor integrative function between the bones of the face, especially those that house the teeth. There were also various restrictions between the bones of the cranial base, so that the brain did not have the space to express its inherent motions properly. Michael's birth had been prolonged as his head was not the best of cranial-pelvic 'fits', and it became unduly compressed. This was the first factor in Michael's life to influence the structure and function of the cranial mechanics. After that had followed a number of sports injuries, childhood illnesses, and falls from his bicycle. Michael's body was resilient and remarkably accommodating, even to the many knocks he'd taken during rugby. But with puberty came structural changes to the fast-growing body and a huge uptake of energy. When the orthodontic appliances were fitted, unfortunately the cranium and its structures were unable to adapt to the added forces, and finally destabilized. The altered cranium placed further forces against the body's resistance and finally the brain's function became altered.

Dental problems have no respect for age. Cutting the first teeth is a painful process which stresses the whole body and is often accompanied by dribbling, a runny nose or a cold. With second teeth come problems of alignment, the height of teeth or overcrowding, which affect the bite. Sometimes specialist orthodontic or dental orthopaedic treatment becomes necessary. These procedures require a child to wear braces, night splints or headgear to move and straighten the teeth or alter the relationships of the upper and lower jaws. As we get older, gum disease may further destabilize the structure and function of the teeth.

The way our teeth function is determined by various factors. We inherit our bone structure and dental predisposition, whilst the quality of food we eat and exposure to different chemicals affects the strength of the teeth and gums. Teeth are also affected by our behavioural patterns, so that when we are anxious or taxing the body there may be an unconscious tendency to grind or clench them.

The skull is a dynamic complex capable of over one hundred articulations through which micro-movements occur. Teeth are extensions of the upper and lower jawbones and articulate directly (or with just one intervening bone) with every other bone in the head. Each tooth forms an articulating joint with the two maxillary bones above and the mandible below which in turn articulates with the two temporal bones to form the jaw joints. The bones of the cranial base can become distorted during the process of birth, and this is reflected through facial asymmetry, at the levels of the eyes or ears. The relationship between the bones influences the position and comfort of the erupting teeth. As teeth make contact, the height of the mouth will affect the position of the jaws. The height is affected by improper eruption of teeth, oral habits and, later, by dental procedures. Habits such as thumb sucking, for example, can affect the way the bones of the mouth mould and so influence the position and health of the teeth.

Teeth tend to move throughout our lives and constantly adapt in a homeostatic balance to the bite. Chewing and swallowing are essential but bring about strong persistent forces on the developing face, transmitted through teeth and via the jaw muscles to the bones of the cranium. So an improper bite will have a detrimental effect on the developing cranium. Developmental stresses imposed on the growing face can influence the future dental pattern. If an osteopath sees children from a young age, she can to some extent predict their future dental mechanics by observing the direction of the growing forces.

When dental appliances are added to a cranium that has unresolved birth strain or compression from injuries, they inhibit the motion of the individual cranial bones. The devices to correct the upper teeth can restrict the inherent motion of the maxillary bones relative to each other, and the bones of the palate. Therefore as the bite changes it strains the relationship of the total cranial mechanism. Headgear can further limit the occipital bones and its relationships to other bones, membranes, cranial nerves and venous drainage. As a result, the face may end up working in one phase of primary respiration whilst the rest of the head works in the opposite phase of motion, which is disharmonious. So, when major dental alterations are made on top of strained cranial mechanics and underlying general stress loads on the body (through puberty, exams or accidents) the coping capacity of the total body system may become compromised. The appliance then becomes the final factor that upsets a delicately balanced system – and headaches, dizziness, irritability, gum soreness or, in Michael's case, where there was an inherent predisposition, symptoms of neurological disturbance may result.

Often in these cases, the teeth may gradually wander back to their previous strained pattern once the corrective dental appliances are removed. But if the underlying problems are corrected before dental therapy starts, any changes to the dental mechanics will occur with greater ease. The orthodontist needs only to encourage the bones and teeth to grow into anatomic relationships which they are ready to accept. In turn, there are fewer side effects and the dental alterations introduced do not degrade once the appliances are removed. The rest of the cranial mechanism adapts more easily to change, the corrected bite remains stable, and it's likely that the dental correction programme will be easier, less uncomfortable and of a shorter duration.

JENNY'S TEETH

The impact of osteopathic work on the jaw and teeth struck me after seeing a series of similar problems. Jenny's is a typical presentation. She was in her forties and suffering with facial pain and a stiff, clicking jaw. Jenny had a poor bite and she clenched her teeth while asleep. She also had occasional headaches, sinusitis and chronic pain in the neck and shoulders. Over a period of time, she had suffered various bouts of ringing in the ears, dizziness, poor eye focusing and fatigue.

After her second treatment, a tooth fell out. I was astonished to hear of this side effect. She laughingly assured me that I had saved her a trip to the dentist since this had been a dying tooth. The same thing happened after the next treatment. Jenny had been through a lot of dental work, including fillings, crowns and root canal therapy, and so the height of the teeth became affected. This variance in height caused the jaws to become misaligned and the overall effect added to pre-existing restrictions within the cranium. The improper relationship of the upper and lower jaws also affected their muscles. For a muscle to work well it must have an optimal length – but, as the height of Jenny's teeth and positions of the jaw altered, the length of the muscles changed, leaving them irritated. This eventually led to chronic facial pain. The seemingly unrelated symptoms of dizziness and equilibrium were due to the altered function of the temporal bones, which house the structures of balance. Because of restricted motion through the maxillary bones and other bones that form the sinuses, Jenny's face could not drain properly and so became reinfected. Her body's unconscious way of relieving stress was to clench her teeth during sleep and as a result the muscles of the head, neck and shoulders were constantly tense, adding to her overall fatigue.

Although Jenny came with facial pain, her treatment programme addressed the whole body and that also included her posture. In the upright position, the body's centre of balance is just behind the jaw. The heavy cranium housing the brain weighs about 4–6 kg (9–14 lb) and is delicately balanced on several flexible vertebrae of the neck. The mandible provides the counterbalance to the skull and its strong muscles and ligaments are attached to the head, face and the neck. Its axis of movement is through the upper two neck vertebrae, so there is constant dialogue between the mouth, the head, and the spinal structures. As a result, the jaw plays an important role in the overall posture of the body and when it loses its place of equilibrium the rest of the body is automatically affected. This can also work the other way, and problems in the pelvis or the spine can affect the jaw position because of the shared stress load from the muscles of the head and neck. This is often seen in people who are too tired to maintain a good posture. When reading a book or watching television, they will often hold their head to support it, which disturbs the balance through the head and jaw.

The treatment approach in most cases of dental and jaw difficulties is to ease out the strain patterns within the head and face bones. This involves balancing the mechanics of the face and jaw in relation to the teeth, the cranium and the rest of the body. This disperses the unconscious need to release tension through clenching and teeth grinding. In Jenny, it seems that as her face and jaw became more efficient, her body rejected the dying teeth. But it is more usual to see this phenomenon the other way round, especially in children. Where a tooth has taken a knock severe enough to affect its blood supply, it is left discoloured and shaky. Encouraging the correct relationship of the tooth with its bone, nerve and blood supply can quickly be done, and can often save the tooth.

Where there are recurrent infections of the teeth or gums, which are not brought about through a lack of hygiene or poor nutrition, correcting the mechanics of the head, face and the neck can help. By removing the restrictions to the drainage mechanisms and nerve, lymph and blood channels, hypersensitivity in the mouth is greatly eased.

5: Backaches and spinal problems

Pain in some region of the spine is by far the most common reason for people to seek help from an osteopath. In the neck, this may also be associated with headaches and perhaps some symptoms in the arm. Although the body has successfully evolved and adapted to being upright, our spines have difficulty with the postural demands we make of them: most problems of the back occur while stooping or standing. Whether at work or travelling, we seem to spend hours bending down, and we often pay a price for this through altered weight-bearing in the spinal structures. However, many things can affect posture – anxiety about deadlines, unhappy relationships, feelings of inadequacy or rejection also influence how we carry ourselves. Often this extra tension is maintained during sleep and we wake not feeling fully restored.

It is very rare for pain to arise for no apparent reason and there is usually a history of previous problems buried somewhere in the tissues. Often this is not alluded to straight away as it is long forgotten, but the effects of previous physical stress stored in the body come to light with each session. The osteopath can usually pick up this information through her dialogue with your tissues. Some of these old stress patterns that weaken the mechanical structures of the spine may go as far back as childhood, with 'growing pains', accidents, infections or illnesses or even old sports injuries.

There are many shades of spinal problems, ranging from the odd stiff back to the severe back pain associated with weakness in the leg or difficulty with urination. This is because there are many types of tissues involved, which behave differently. The stiff back may result from tense muscles, while the severe pain might be due to a prolapsed disc pressing on the spinal cord. Some soft tissue release and gentle manipulation to increase mobility at the spinal restrictions might be sufficient to treat the stiffness. On the other hand, a severely prolapsed disc with complications will need an operation to release the pressure on the spinal cord.

Efficient spinal mechanics are dictated by how well the ligaments and soft tissues support the vertebral column. In a balanced posture, bones at strategic areas of the body take the compressive forces of gravity and weight bearing. The centre of gravity in the body is a theoretical point in space that falls in front of the sacrum. Because it is so far up from the ground the potential for mobility and movement in the human body is great, but it is precisely because of this that we are inherently unstable. There is a high potential for the soft tissue spinal support to become weak, especially in the standing position, because when the gravity centre shifts, demands are placed on structures that are not designed for weight bearing. As the spinal support provided by the membranous tensional network erodes, the vertebral joints become too mobile and unstable,

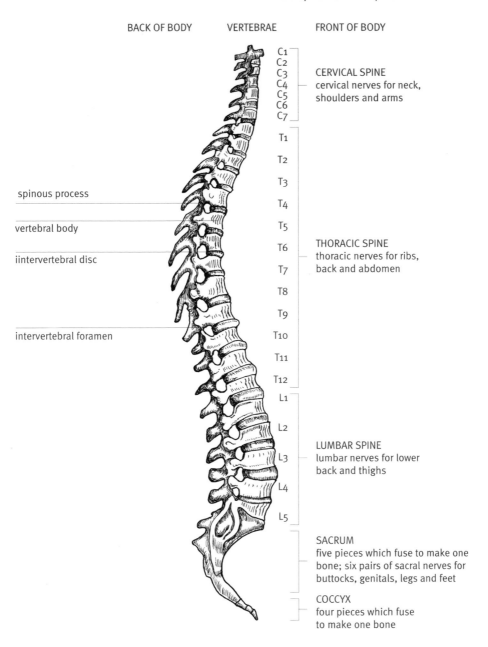

Figure 8 THE VERTEBRAL COLUMN AND SPINAL NERVES
Side view showing natural curves. Spinal nerves leave
the spinal column in pairs on either side of the spine.

BACK OF BODY   VERTEBRAE   FRONT OF BODY

C1
C2
C3   CERVICAL SPINE
C4   cervical nerves for neck,
C5   shoulders and arms
C6
C7

T1
T2
T3
T4
spinous process
T5
vertebral body
T6   THORACIC SPINE
            thoracic nerves for ribs,
iintervertebral disc   T7   back and abdomen
T8
T9
intervertebral foramen   T10
T11
T12
L1
L2
            LUMBAR SPINE
L3   lumbar nerves for lower
            back and thighs
L4
L5

SACRUM
five pieces which fuse to make one
bone; six pairs of sacral nerves for
buttocks, genitals, legs and feet

COCCYX
four pieces which fuse
to make one bone

For a chart showing the spinal segments and their
inter-relationships with the body parts, see appendix 1.

The vertebral column contains the spinal cord as it
exits from the foramen magnum of the cranium. It
carries the spinal cord, and spinal nerves leave the
column in pairs on either side of the spine through the
intervertebral foramen There is one pair of spinal nerves
for each vertebral segment, except at the tail end.

93

Figure 9 A CROSS-SECTION OF A DAMAGED VERTEBRAL SEGMENT

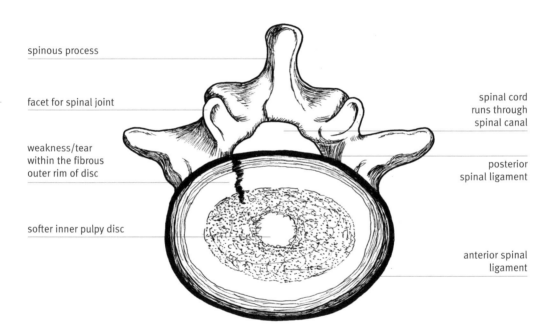

BACK OF BODY

spinous process

facet for spinal joint

weakness/tear
within the fibrous
outer rim of disc

softer inner pulpy disc

spinal cord
runs through
spinal canal

posterior
spinal ligament

anterior spinal
ligament

FRONT OF BODY

The soft pulpy nucleus at the centre of the disc may bulge on to the weakness in the fibrous outer rim of the disc. Eventually this bulge may be large enough to cause pressure on the pain-sensitive spinal ligament, and also on the spinal nerve. If the outer rim is too weak, it may result in the prolapse of the pulpy nucleus.

Figure 10 INVERTEBRAL FORAMEN
View of two lumbar vertebrae side on to show spinal
nerves leaving the vertebral canal

intervertebral foramen

spinal nerve root –
pierces the spinal
membrane (dura)
within the foramen
before exiting

body of vertebra

intervertebral disc

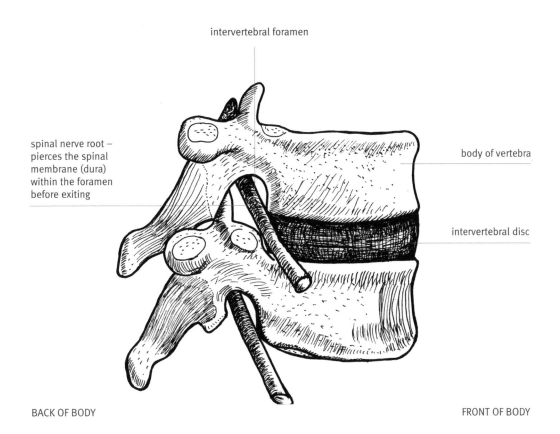

BACK OF BODY

FRONT OF BODY

usually at the lower lumbar and cervical areas. In turn, other vertebral joints become more restricted and the biomechanics of the spine become compromised so that weight is unevenly taken on the intervertebral discs.

Each disc lies between a pair of vertebrae and it must retain its structural integrity in order to function normally. It might help to think of the structure of a disc as a tyre. The strong external fibrous layer of the disc is like a tyre's outer hard rubber ring, while the pulpy nucleus inside the disc is akin to the soft and compressible inner tube. A defect in the outer section of the tyre may have various causes, such as a manufacturing flaw, wear and tear or hitting the kerb suddenly. A weakness is then created in the outer rim. The pressure within the inner tube pushes on this weakness in the outer rim, so that it starts to bulge and, over time, will burst. Similarly, the weakness of the outer fibrous component of the disc may be due to a genetic defect, degeneration, nutritional deficiency or trauma. The pressure within the nucleus pulposis, the central part of the disc, acts on this area so that it bulges, with symptoms of aching and stiffness. The rim eventually ruptures with extrusion of the disc material, and as this encroaches on the space of the vertebral canal it irritates the pain-sensitive ligaments lining the spinal column. This generally occurs through wear and tear, sometimes exacerbated by a sudden additional load, as in lifting weight, or in a sudden act, such as coughing. The protruding disc material can in turn press on to the nerve emerging from the spinal cord, which gives pain, pins and needles, numbness, and if severe enough, reduces the strength of either the arm or the leg, depending on the area affected. (See figure 9.)

JORG'S BACK

Jorg was suffering. He arrived bent to the side and each movement felt like a lightning seizure in his lower back, sending pain down the right leg. The intensity of pain made Jorg very tense and apprehensive. He prayed he would not sneeze. The pain gored into the back, and was now spreading upwards towards the neck. He barely managed to doze at night, taking a combination of strong painkillers and muscle relaxants. Morning was the worst time; he felt 'locked', and it took a good twenty minutes of rocking to and fro before he felt remotely mobile. Jorg had always enjoyed good health and his back only became troublesome when he moved home three months ago. However, this had not bothered him until ten days previously when his back just gave way as he reached down to pick up some files.

He had difficulty performing any movements, and was only able to move the upper part of his body. All the tendon reflexes were within normal limits. However, lying on his back and raising his right leg to just 30 degrees worsened the pain, indicating nerve involvement. MRI scans had revealed two bulging discs, the worst one being at the spinal junction with the pelvis. This had herniated to the right, irritating the sciatic nerve down the leg; not bad enough to operate, but still nasty. In trying to adapt and respond to the damage in the disc, Jorg's body automatically attempted to take the weight off it, causing him to be all bent up.

Treating Jorg was complicated; his only comfortable position was lying on his side. There was a palpable sense of 'bogginess' in the tissues of the lower back, indicative of the swelling and congestion there. Overlying this, spasm could be felt in the deep muscles as they tried to protect the disc from herniating further. The treatment plan required a double strategy. In the short term, he needed help with the pain and mobility by taking the extra load off the lower spine and so reducing the inflammation. In the long term, however, his body's tensional network needed to be re-established so that the weight would be more evenly distributed throughout the whole spine, rather than at a few levels. This meant altering the mechanics of the entire spine, and balancing the cranium and pelvis as well as the relationships of the legs to enable lasting stability.

When I felt Jorg's back, the motions of primary respiration seemed to be restricted in the lower part of the back. The last two vertebrae seemed to be compressed together, squeezing the disc. And where it had herniated on to the space where the spinal nerve exits the vertebral canal, it created a kink in the curtain of the dural membranes, setting up interference to the normal tidal motions at this level. This was resonating in the neck as well. Gently separating the last two vertebral bones and the sacrum reduced extra compression on them and eased the pressure off the disc. The muscles were allowed to lengthen to enable the disc more space to find its own position of balance, whilst nudging the vertebral bones towards the middle axis of the body. In so doing, the venous and lymphatic drainage was enhanced and the congestion was reduced. This gradually released the pressure of the nerve root, thereby easing the pain in the leg. By cradling the cranium and the sacrum, the tension within the membranes lining the spinal cord and nerve were gently allowed to alter their point of balance through their bony attachments.

After the first two sessions, Jorg managed to sleep and the angry pain began to subside. The structural integrity of the disc pulp and its fibrous rim was improved by coaxing them towards a balanced central axis. After about three weeks he had made a 60 per cent recovery and his mobility gradually increased. As Jorg had stooped to pick up the files, the forces of leverage through the spine, right arm and leg became concentrated on to the level of the herniated disc. As the compressive forces of these vectors were released, the quality and range of spinal motion started to get smoother.

Although he got back to his normal routine, two months later some long drives made Jorg's back ache and his leg was occasionally annoying. As Jorg lay on his back, I felt a sense of tightness at the level of the waist, at the right psoas muscle. This tension must have been there for some time, probably from an old injury, sending reflex tightness towards the pelvis. With one hand on the lower back, and the other at the abdomen, the tension in these tissues was unwound. As this was happening, Jorg experienced intense pain in his leg, which demanded attention. So I placed one hand on the right knee while the other remained under Jorg's back so the thigh could be balanced with the spine and pelvis and the nerve circuit between the spinal cord and the leg was retuned. This produced a dramatic shift in the way Jorg's body regained its function.

Many factors play their part in the maintenance of poor health and spinal function. Because the spine is so heavily loaded with nerves, a mechanical irritation of a nerve means it is continually stressed and borders on a state of alarm. Therefore, even mild stimulation, such as might occur in moving suddenly, causes the emergency reflex to approach maximum activity rapidly. Also, 'chatter' between segments up and down the spinal highway means that areas remote from the irritated segment can become additional locations for pain. Such impulses can also be sent into the organs and internal structures, so feelings of excessive sweating, nausea, poor appetite or disturbed bowel function are common with back pain.

Many biomechanical and biochemical factors will also contribute to the make-up of the spine. Genetic predisposition to joint problems, family history of arthritis, or diabetes, poor nutrition and even excessive alcohol and smoking will all affect the overall quality of the body's tissues. These leave a sense of rigidity and fatigue that affects the tissues making up the support of the spinal column and the disc material. Wear and tear is accelerated when combined with repeated physical work, especially in damp conditions. The treatment then must be thought of in terms of months, and is aimed at re-establishing stability and co-ordination through the spinal tensional network and improving the quality of the tissues through encouraging fluid interchange. This can be assisted by self-help measures such as changes in diet, which help to harmonize the pH balance of the tissues. In general acid foods should be avoided. Nutritional supplements such as glucosamine phosphate and herbal remedies may also be recommended.

Chapter five

Pregnancy and childbirth

Every woman comes . . . with a unique personal, family and cultural history that will strongly influence the course of her labour . . . A woman brings to childbirth her entire life experience, reaching as far back as her own infancy and birth.

Michel Odent

Osteopathy was inspired by children, for it was after Dr Still tragically lost his children to meningitis that he began his search into the nature of health and disease.

We know that the future health of the developing child will be influenced by the physical and emotional wellbeing of the parents. However, many chronic health problems can be attributed to the effects of pregnancy and labour. Osteopaths who work with children therefore see the treatment of the new mother as being crucial. Within the first few months, the baby also thinks of himself as an extension of the mother, so the treatment of the newborn is likely to be more effective if the mother also receives attention. In this chapter I will be looking at pregnancy and childbirth both from the perspective of the expectant mother and that of the developing child. The mother will be considered first.

Pregnancy

Pregnancy is a time of phenomenal transformation where the mother will experience a myriad of emotional, physical, chemical and hormonal changes. The expectant mother's body is constantly adapting to accommodate the growing baby, deliver that baby and then, remarkably, restore itself. If, however there have been some pre-existing problems affecting the back or the pelvis, the expectant mother's body may not adapt to these changes. At this time, the osteopath can assist by restoring and improving the overall function of her body. As she becomes free of any restrictions and undue strains, she can more readily adapt to the demands of pregnancy and birth.

Pregnancy is accompanied by postural adaptations, which occur in response to the growing uterus. The enlarging abdomen causes the weight of the body to tip forwards so that the lower spine becomes hollow. The body accommodates this swayback posture by releasing hormones to soften the ligaments of the spine and pelvis, so they are not strained. However, if the network of ligaments and membranes is already weakened or there is poor abdominal tone, then the body may not be able to adapt so well to the new changes. A variety of symptoms may be felt, depending on the area of strain, but lower backache is most common. As the neck and shoulders become rounded, headaches or pins and needles in the arms from irritated nerves and blood vessels can also occur. Nausea, breathlessness, fatigue, heartburn, constipation, piles and varicose veins are common in pregnancy and most of these symptoms are related to the way the muscles, spine, nerves and circulatory channels accommodate the changing size, shape and weight of the uterus. Sometimes, the baby can lie awkwardly and irritate the sciatic nerve, giving pain in the leg. Pressure from the baby on organs and their connected fascias, nerves, blood and lymphatic channels contribute to some of the above symptoms, but most of them disappear with birth.

Most expectant mothers can manage some level of discomfort, seeing it as part of the process – but when there have been previous problems, the body may have difficulty in coping with the changes of pregnancy. The size and shape of the pelvis, trouble with a previous labour, scarring, injuries or illnesses alter the ability of the pelvis to accommodate the growing baby and ultimately affect his passage through the birth canal. Often, the treatment is to gently enable the body to adapt to postural changes. The sacrum is encouraged to find a position of ease within the pelvis and this helps the spine since the body weight becomes more central. The spinal joints and ribs can get very stiff and so affect the autonomic nerve pathways, causing reflex tension in the stomach and the gut. Treatment is aimed at maintaining the expectant mother's posture, spinal and pelvic mechanics so that she is comfortable and so the pelvic bones can easily separate for the passage of the baby during labour.

Childbirth

Just as each pregnancy is unique, so too is each birth. Although labour is very painful it is often 'forgotten' relatively quickly – the mother has to get on with looking after her baby and her own physical and emotional needs can get overlooked. Even mothers who have had a Caesarean section may not really acknowledge to themselves that they have had an operation. In traditional African and Indian village communities, it is common for the extended family or neighbours to help in the care of the new mother and child. There is often a period of time, usually forty days, when the mother is supported with massage and energy-giving foods to aid recovery and allow bonding time with the baby. But in modern Western society this is almost impossible – the mother usually returns home with little support or post-natal care, to juggle with domestic tasks, new family dynamics and managing her career as well.

Having to cope with all this, the new mother places herself low on her list of priorities. Yet during the process of labour her whole being, and certainly her body, has undergone a marathon. The labour position, the baby's presenting position, the type of painkilling agent, as well as the emotional experience of it all, will contribute to the effects of labour. Any unresolved stresses and strains on her body may lead to a slumped posture with back pain, fatigue, incontinence, mood swings and a loss of libido, which may not present until some time later. The osteopath will often feel a sense of heaviness throughout the body, almost as if everything needs to be lifted back upwards.

During the process of labour, the sacrum, coccyx and the pelvic bones spread slightly apart under the influence of the softened ligaments to make space for the passage of the baby. Within about six weeks of delivery, the hormones diminish so that the ligaments resume their tone, the bones return to their normal position, the extended abdomen recedes and the posture gradually returns. However, the altered relationship of the various parts of the pelvis may not resolve completely. The baby's emerging head can often exert a great deal of pressure on any of the pelvic bones and the attached soft tissues so that pressure on the sacrum, for example, may upset its relationship with the coccyx. During second stage labour, the mother's pelvis has already separated as much as it can. The use of forceps can sometimes further stress the mother's pelvis beyond the elastic capacity of the ligaments and soft tissues. This means that as the ligaments tighten again after the birth when realignment is taking place, the pelvic bones and attached soft tissues remain in an unbalanced and strained position. This can predispose to problems within the pelvis and prevent posture from reverting to normal.

ANNA'S ACCIDENTS

Anna looked drained, was pale and felt low. She had been having 'accidents' when she could not immediately get to the toilet. Coughing and sneezing resulted in urinary incontinence, which started after the birth of Peter five years ago. Prior to that she used to get cramps with periods, but over the last three years, she had got headaches instead. As this was her first pregnancy, Anna did not seem a likely candidate for this sort of incontinence problem, so there must have been some underlying factors. As a teenager, Anna rode a horse and remembered falling on to the coccyx and being sore for weeks. Within a year she had an appendectomy.

During the latter part of the pregnancy, the baby had lain low and Anna had suffered with pain at the front of the pelvis. This is where the two bones of the pelvis meet to form a joint, the pubic symphysis, and the ligaments were strained. During labour, Anna was given an epidural injection for the pain, but because the labour had become prolonged she needed medication to increase the contractions. After a number of hours, Anna had difficulty pushing because she was so exhausted. Finally, both ventous(a suction device similar to a sink plunger) and forceps were used to extract the baby. Anna was very fatigued, had back pain and did not leave the hospital for eight days.

On examining Anna, I found there was little energy in her tissues, which felt ropey. She still had the swayback posture and the pelvic bones had not resumed their normal position after the birth. The sacrum felt unstable and unsupported by the ligaments; its relationship with the coccyx must initially have been altered by falling off her horse and was worsened by giving birth. The motion of the sacrum was restricted and the attached soft tissues and membranes of the pelvic floor felt equally strained and sagging. This had prevented the bladder from returning to its normal position so that its function was altered. There was also a dragging sensation through the spinal membranes, felt throughout the body right up into the cranial membranes.

Osteopaths find that it is important to treat the effects of an epidural, as when the body is already compensating for previous problems recovery may be affected. The epidural injection into the spinal dural membrane numbs the nerves to the uterus. Ordinarily the mother would respond to pain and pressure by moving out of the position of strain. However, with an epidural she is required to stay still and does not feel the excessive stretch and pressure on her back and pelvis. In addition, there will be a micro-scar at the injection site which, as Anna already had a pelvic problem, helped to maintain the hollow back.

During labour Anna was bearing down with such force that with each contraction the uterus, diaphragm, neck, shoulders and even her face strained to give birth to the baby. Eventually she could not synchronize the push with the contractions and, as a result, the rhythms of the diaphragm and the uterus got confused. The downward pressure from the baby on the sacrum dragged it to a position lower than normal, leaving it unable to move freely between the pelvic bones. This not only affected Anna's spinal and pelvic mechanics, but the related nerves and pelvic organs as well. The consequence was a weakness of the pelvic floor and the ligaments that support the bladder, resulting in stress incontinence. Anna was also feeling low. Although post-natal depression is thought to be a hormonal problem, its mechanical causes may stem from unresolved birth strain. The drag from the sacrum and coccyx carries into the cranium because of the spinal and cranial membranes. Bearing in mind these membranes also cover the brain and spinal cord, the effect is to create a pull on the brain and the pituitary gland, which can result in an altered function of the hormonal system. In addition, because there is a lot of emotional instability, especially fear, at the time of birth, the nervous system engraves this into the body tissues so that the muscles tense up.

Anna's treatment was directed mainly at restoring the function of the pelvis and the structures contained in it. As the pelvic bones and their soft tissues were restored to their natural state, the bladder gradually returned to its normal position. The pelvic floor muscles and ligaments could now support the bladder and Anna maintained their tone through exercises. When the sacrum could move freely the tension in the membranes eased and this took the slack off the brain and spinal cord, so hormonal balance could return. Restoring the harmony between the diaphragm and the pelvic floor muscles re-established the normal breathing pattern and the function of the abdomen and, overall, Anna's vitality improved.

The baby during pregnancy

The womb is the baby's first world and his development there may be affected in many ways. The structure and function of the developing foetus is susceptible to mechanical, nutritional and environmental influences whose effects may show only in later life. High blood pressure in mid-life, for example, has been attributed to the ratio of the birthweight with that of the placenta, and is directly related to the status of the foetus at 4–20 weeks of gestation. The way the baby experiences the womb may predispose personality and character. In *The Secret Life of the Unborn Child* Verny and Kelly describe how sounds, voices and other factors shape the physical and emotional health of the baby. A safe uterine world may encourage confidence in the outside world, while the uterus might seem like a hostile environment to a baby who experiences distress or unexpected heavy bleeding (perhaps as a result of placental problems).

Severe maternal distress, such as the death of someone deeply loved, or other influences such as exposure to chemicals, are known to affect the structural development of the baby. But other, subtler, effects may also be related to the baby's ability to cope with the stresses of birth.

With the decline in the extended family system, there is often little support for the mother in terms of housework, preparing meals, and the emotional buffers so needed at this time. An unplanned pregnancy, a toddler in tow, insecurities around a new job, difficult relationships, moving home or building work may in themselves be manageable, but none the less bring additional stress. Although most people get through these difficulties somehow, if the mother's feelings of prolonged anxiety are accompanied with inadequate rest, poor nutrition and domestic support, the baby's response to stress may be heightened. Although each has a separate nervous and blood circulatory system, the mother and her developing baby hold a dialogue through the nervous and hormonal links. This is especially the case on an emotional level so that if the mother is distressed, her stress neuro-hormones cross the placenta. It is not known at which point the developing baby's brain is most vulnerable to these maternal overflows, but it seems that the hypothalamus may become particularly sensitive. When the levels of stress neuro-hormones remain raised in the mother over a period of time, these levels gradually become the norm for the developing baby. In turn, this can affect his ability to cope with future distress.

During birth, the baby releases very high levels of stress neuro-hormones, especially when the delivery is complicated. They are needed to produce energy, afford protection from any lack of oxygen and prepare for survival outside the womb. Usually these settle down shortly after birth. As we have just seen, however, where there has been maternal distress the baby's stress response has already been pre-set to a higher level, leaving fewer reserves to counter the effects of birth. The osteopath feels this as excessive tension throughout the body, which in turn makes the baby behave as if constantly 'on alert'. He startles easily, is irritable or clingy. Prolonged stress in the adult is known to affect the immune system. In babies exposed to maternal distress and a complicated birth there seems to be a predisposition to recurrent infections and allergies, especially when there is a family history of allergy. Treatment in these cases is as much aimed at supporting the immune function as helping the body to deal with the unresolved effects of stress.

The dialogue between the mother and the baby is physiological as well as emotional. At the time of birth, the mother's pelvis responds to the emerging baby by expanding and in turn the shape of the baby's head changes so that he can negotiate his way into the world. As life inside the uterus ends, life in the outside world is just beginning.

The impact of labour on the baby's cranium

MATTHEW'S BIRTH

Matthew was just three weeks old; his face was paralysed on one side. There was a degree of floppiness about him and yet, paradoxically, there was also a feeling of immense tightness within his whole being. He had not been able to feed from the breast but was a calm and placid baby, crying gently only when hungry or wet.

Jean had easily carried Matthew to term, but had not been prepared for the rather traumatic events of birth. The contractions kept coming strong and hard but nothing seemed to happen. Matthew was stuck, unable to get his head past a certain point, no matter how hard Jean pushed. Finally, he was delivered using ventouse and forceps. He emerged blue, exhausted and limp; his head was misshapen and his face was bruised. He did not breathe and needed to be resuscitated. He was whisked away to the special care baby unit, where he stayed for the next week. During this time Matthew's condition improved, but he still remained relatively floppy, dribbled and found feeding difficult. Matthew was diagnosed with possible cerebral palsy.

Watching Matthew, I noticed that only the left side of the face crinkled as he cried, while the other side remained smooth. Crying was such an effort that he was left exhausted. On feeling him, I noticed a striking sense of shock throughout his body. This was apparent not only in the circulatory system but also through the sense of a sudden, traumatic disturbance to the physical and emotional equilibrium. It was felt in both rigidity and inertia of the tissues, which seemed frozen. The membranes and bones at the base of the skull, especially on the right side, felt taut and compressed. The vault bones overlapped and felt out of sync with their counterparts at the base of the skull and the face, so that the brain felt cramped. The rhythmic motion of the brain and its fluid felt restrained, matching the restrictions of the cranium. The shape of the face reflected its having been squashed in the narrow part of Jean's pelvis and this was even carried through to the upper part of the neck. Matthew's chest felt tight and his breathing was laboured. Surprisingly, however, under this feeling of shock and in spite of the structural and mechanical problems, Matthew's overall vitality and constitution felt very strong.

Matthew's treatment was geared to taking the shock out of his system and reinstating the rhythmic motion. To give the brain more space to work, the compression at the base of the skull and the tension within the cranial membranes was released. As Matthew had tried to come out face first the head kept jamming up against the tight wall of the cervix with the force of each contraction. In addition, the weight of the descending body added to the forces placed on the head and neck. Ideally, the baby has the resources to allow the bones of the skull to realign after birth. Unfortunately Matthew's head and face were so squashed by the compressive forces of labour and he was so exhausted that the bones and membranes could not find that balance. Once this was allowed to happen, the brain function began to improve and the paralysed side of the face started to crease up as Matthew cried. The odd thing now was that the opposite side, originally thought to be normal, did not crease up as much as the other side! This revealed the true extent of the paralysis, which had, in effect, been bilateral, but worse on the right. As the tension was released from the chest and diaphragm, an even, rhythmic breath began to permeate the body. The emotional shock began to lift and as the communication between the brain and the body improved so too did the mobility of his limbs.

Matthew responded well, needing only a few treatments as he had such good vitality. By the time he was a year old the face was creasing up on both sides as he laughed. The floppiness had virtually gone, to be replaced by a much healthier overall tone in his body and he could function well under his own steam.

To understand why Matthew ended up with problems after his protracted journey through the birth canal, it is useful to see what happens during the normal process of birth. The baby usually lies upside down, with the head leading the way. The muscular walls of the uterus undergo very powerful contractions, pushing the baby down the birth canal. The head undergoes various positional changes so that maximum space within the pelvic cavity can be gained. This ensures that the widest part of the head corresponds to the widest diameter of the pelvis at the time of exit. For any part of the body to grow and function efficiently it must have adequate space to express its motion, just as the roots of a plant need a spacious enough pot. It is therefore necessary that the container – the body structure – is kept free of any restrictions. This is especially important for the central nervous system, since much of its growth and development occurs after birth.

The emerging baby can easily accommodate the intense pressures of this journey because of the design of the cranium. It is malleable, has the ability to bend and distort and yet is sufficiently strong to protect the delicate brain and spinal cord. While it can adapt to the enormous compressive forces of labour, it is also elastic enough to recover from these after the birth.

Because of the way it is structured, the skull is sufficiently pliable for passage through the birth canal, where it undergoes changes in shape and size. The bones or plates of the vault develop within a continuous membrane with six wide spaces or fontanelles separating them, which accounts for their flexibility and the ability to overlap in response to the compressive forces of labour. After birth, as the baby grows, the plates expand outwards so that the soft fontanelles gradually close up to form sutures, where motion between the neighbouring bones can occur.

The bones at the base of the cranium are partly made from cartilage, the same flexible structure as is found in the nose. An important aspect of these stiffer bones at the cranial base is that some of them consist of more than one part: this allows hinging between the component parts and means that they can bend and warp. Usually when a child is between three and nine years old, the component parts fuse to make a single bone.

Of these bones in the cranial base, the occipital bone at the back of the head has particular importance at birth. It is made from four distinct areas so that minute motion can be accommodated within them to enable the cranium to adapt to the forces of birth. The occipital bone also defines the shape of the space (the foramen magnum) for the transition between the brain and spinal cord running through it. Therefore a twist or distortion between the parts can impose restriction on the movement of this very important structure. The temporal and sphenoid bones are similarly formed in three separate parts and also allow distortion. Gradually, the bones of the skull harden in a process that is not complete until around the age of 25.

Cranial moulding and birth compression

During birth the tissues reflect the compression forces of labour and the shape of the head changes. When this is extreme, the structures within the skull may not adapt well to the relatively sudden changes. The resulting pull on the cranial membranes can distort the blood vessels contained in them and also affect the nerves as they exit the cranium.

The head's adjustment to the size and shape of the birth canal is known as cranial moulding. At birth, the baby gets more compressed in order to pass down the birth canal. In the majority of deliveries, the distortions correct within a few hours to days, thanks to the forces of crying, breathing, yawning and suckling. As the skull expands, so the changes in the shape of the head become noticeable and the baby settles. The process of birth is the biggest stress that we undergo in our lives and the effort required is phenomenal. The baby has to adapt to the mother's pelvis and accept the compression forces of labour. Having emerged, he has to expend yet more energy to resolve these compressive forces and set in motion what he now needs to survive in the outside world. The first breath starts these processes by expanding the lungs and switching on the breathing mechanics. The breath will open up air spaces for the first time and in so doing animate every single cell in the body. In turn, the body opens and spreads. As the baby cries and yawns, the cranial base and vault release their compression and expand fully, whilst the bodily movements release compression strains in the pelvis, spine and the entire body. When the baby suckles the palate and tongue work to mobilize rhythmically all the tissues as far as the sacrum and the coccyx. This process of unfolding is visible as the shape of the head changes and the body relaxes, just as a rosebud is seen to bloom. The baby usually settles within about two weeks.

In previous times, in villages of India and Africa, women well versed in the aftereffects of birth would massage and gently press the head in order to 'unmould' the skull bones and assist the resolution of the birth process. They would also massage the newborn's body and limbs, to help with mobility, circulation, breathing and digestion and to encourage the baby's sensitivity to touch. Nowadays these women are a rarity, even in the old village communities, and babies do not have the benefit of this honoured tradition.

Shock

The baby's unfolding process may be inhibited as a result of a labour that is protracted, complicated or even too quick. Although the cranial vault acquires a normal shape, the distortions in the stiffer bones of the base are much harder for the baby to resolve and, as they are beneath the vault, they lie hidden. Shock is a major cause of incomplete unfolding. Both shock and foetal distress have a wider meaning to the osteopath, indicative of the baby's emotional and physiological response when his survival is suddenly threatened. In a complicated delivery the dialogue between the mother and the emerging baby is suddenly disrupted and, in turn, her fears enter the equation. The tissues of the baby reflect this as a motion that feels frozen, as if stunned. As a result the newborn is often either subdued or irritable, will not settle, is wakeful and over-alert or hyper-responsive to sensations. The sense of shock and foetal distress is deeply intertwined: it can be visualized as a rosebud prevented from opening because it has been caught by an unexpected frost. Once released, the tissues can expand and open up more freely.

Birth position

The baby's orientation at birth is an important factor in determining the outcome of labour because of the position of the head relative to the spine. The normal position is where the baby is facing backwards, head down and chin tucked in, known as flexion, and it provides the best cranial-pelvic fit. Other positions may be adopted by the baby, which can complicate the delivery. This is because either the head is not the best fit with the mother's pelvis, or it is not the presenting part. Then the labour is often protracted and the mother gets exhausted, so forceps or ventouse are needed for turning the head or extracting the baby. A common position is with the back against the mother's spine so that as the head descends, it faces forwards and the flexion is poor. Matthew came out that way, and we saw how he got stuck en route. On the other hand, where a baby has been lying transverse, the presenting part is often the shoulder. Extra force may be needed to pull him through and this means that the neck and shoulder area can get strained. In almost a quarter of pregnancies, at the 30th week the baby is in a breech or bottom downward position, which means that many premature births occur in this position. Where the bottom is the presenting part, the pelvis meets the greater part of the compressive forces of labour and also, there is no time for moulding of the head. The osteopath can feel these birth strain patterns through the body tissues.

Problems with cranial nerves

Sometimes unresolved cranial base restriction and compression may interfere with the function of the brain and the emerging cranial nerves (see figure 4). The symptoms depend on which cranial nerve is affected. Difficulty in suckling, for example, can be a direct effect of distortion disturbing the passage of the hypoglossal nerve, which affects suckling, tongue movements and the development of speech. Irritation of the vagus nerve that supplies the gut can be the cause of colic, with the baby being distressed around feeding times.

The compression forces of birth may also affect the abdomen, pelvis and the spine. The baby can get compressed through the spine and this has many implications. If it affects the neck then the baby may favour lying on one side or have difficulty in turning one way; he may yell each time the head is touched, as it can be very sensitive. A common feature is a wry neck or torticollis, where the neck is held on one side. This is usually due to compression inside the womb affecting the sternomastoid muscle at the front of the neck, though distortion and compression within the bones of the cranial base can also affect the attachments of the neck muscles.

Any distortion or compression at the pelvis and sacrum can affect the growth and development of the spine and developing posture. Apart from this, the spine carries the nerves of the autonomic system that supply the organs, so that after a period of time, symptoms may arise depending on which level of the spine is affected. When the nerves to the gut are disturbed, this is echoed as tension in the fascias and the abdomen. Unresolved birth strain can also be found in the abdomen. The gut and intestines will ordinarily expand into any available space in the abdomen and pelvis, but when there is compression it can reduce the space available to the digestive organs. The overall result is a variety of non-specific symptoms such as colic, constipation or wind. The baby is not happy, cannot settle and this in turn leads to problems with sleeping patterns.

Assisted delivery – foetal distress

When the baby cannot progress any further down the birth canal, forceps or ventouse may be used. In a difficult delivery, the head has already undergone as much alteration of its shape as is possible. So, whilst these appliances are life-saving, their use may add to the amount of cranial distortion, which is difficult for the baby to resolve.

In some cases, the delivery is complicated because the umbilical cord is tightly wrapped round the neck. This can compromise the baby's blood supply leading to foetal distress. There are other causes of foetal distress, but the common effect is a shortage of oxygen. The effects on the baby and his development will be mild to severe depending on the degree of shortage. There may be no effects noted at birth, but they may show up later in slight

Figure 11 THE CRANIUM OF A BABY (SHOWING FONTANELLES)

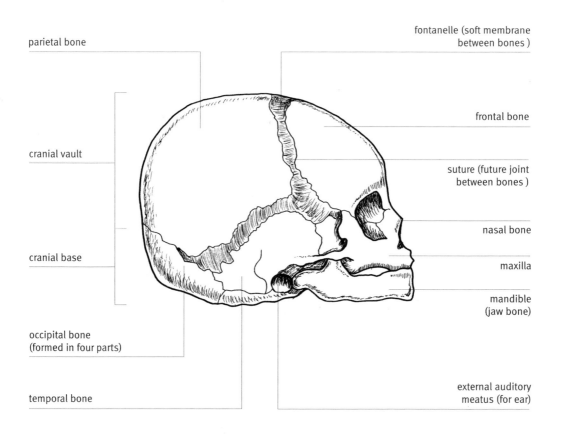

parietal bone

fontanelle (soft membrane between bones)

cranial vault

frontal bone

suture (future joint between bones)

nasal bone

cranial base

maxilla

mandible (jaw bone)

occipital bone (formed in four parts)

temporal bone

external auditory meatus (for ear)

The bones at the top of the skull, or vault bones, are formed by growing in membranes, whilst those at the base of the skull are formed in slightly stiffer cartilage. The bones grow into the membranous spaces, which eventually become sutures or joints between the cranial bones. This flexibility and pliability is especially important for moulding during the birth process.

Figure 12 THE OCCIPITAL BONE AT BIRTH

In a newborn the occipital bone, found at the base of the skull, is in four parts, which functionally act as separate bones that are capable of moving in relation to each other at the time of birth.

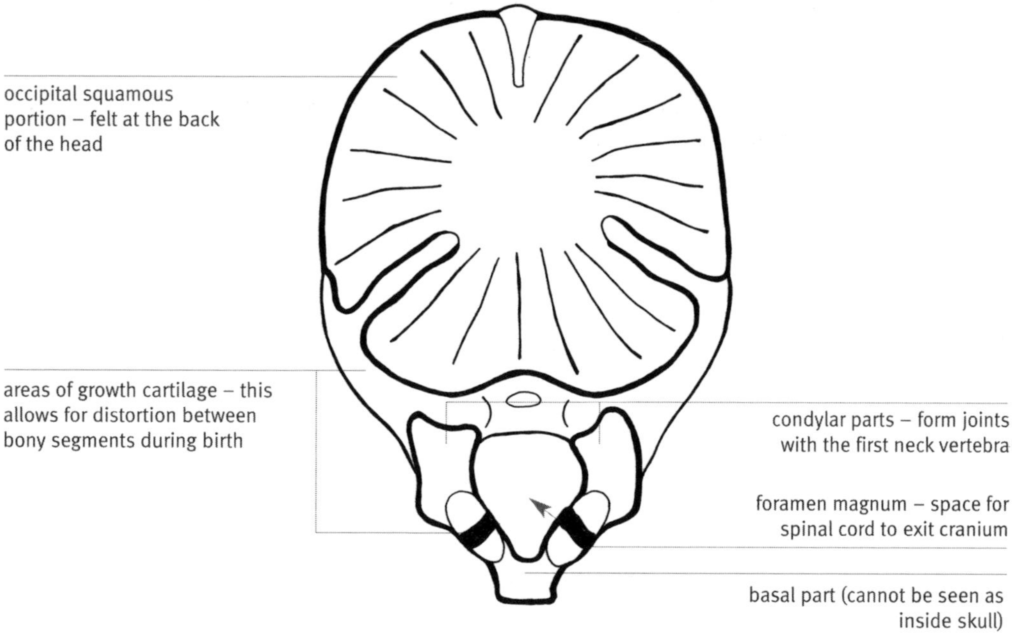

occipital squamous portion – felt at the back of the head

areas of growth cartilage – this allows for distortion between bony segments during birth

condylar parts – form joints with the first neck vertebra

foramen magnum – space for spinal cord to exit cranium

basal part (cannot be seen as inside skull)

Figure 13 DISTORTION OF THE OCCIPITAL BONE
Distortion of the four parts of the occipital bone as a result of birth trauma

Occipital squamous portion has twisted and compressed on to the condylar parts

distortion of the space of foramen magnum

area of compression or distortion

area of distortion and compression on to 1st neck vertebra

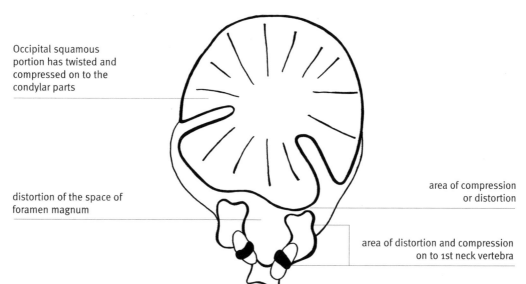

developmental problems. Or there may be overt brain damage. The osteopath feels the nervous system as having a strained and limited rhythmic motion and this is a major factor for the baby who is unable to recover from birth strain, the effects of which remain within the tissues.

Premature babies

Babies born before the 37th week are considered to be premature and their problems will depend on the degree of prematurity and the intervention needed. The main difficulty for the premature baby is the immaturity of the lungs due to a lack of surfactant, a substance that gives elasticity, which is why very premature babies need a ventilator to help them breathe. When a ventilator is used over a period of time, the bones of the head and face mould around this tube. These distinctive features are seen in the shape of the face, whilst the stress within the lungs is felt as a tense and inelastic quality. This can predispose the infant to problems such as infections and asthma. Although the head is smaller than at term, the bones are more soft and pliable; it is therefore particularly vulnerable to the compressive forces of labour and gravity. As a result the head becomes easily flattened when lying on the favoured side. The premature baby can be greatly helped by osteopathy and the treatments are very short and gentle, aimed at supporting the baby's innate health. As shock and strain patterns are released, the baby often becomes visibly more relaxed.

Chapter six

The growing years: children and adolescents

As a twig is bent, so the tree inclines.

Dr William Garner Sutherland

Problems that we suffer as adults often have their beginnings in our early years. Back pain, for example, is currently one of the main reasons for lost working days. Back pain is largely due to some breakdown in the spinal mechanics, but the initial factors that influence the way the spine develops may well be related to retained compressive birth stresses. Many conditions affecting the growing child can be attributed to the secondary effects of retained moulding and birth strain. When not resolved, this stress causes distortions within the tissues to become part of the normal growing physiology. The body adapts and grows around the forces of birth, and early care and attention to the developing structure and function can influence the course of the child's health, providing essential preventive care.

As the baby grows there is a sequence to the acquisition of movement, such as rolling over, sitting up, crawling and so on. When the nervous system, muscle strength and co-ordination are sufficiently developed the child can move on to a new stage. However, not all systems of the body grow at the same pace. Bones grow at different rates, while the brain grows in spurts that begin in the middle of pregnancy and continue until the third year of life. Different types of brain cell have different growth spurts and the process of myelination (the insulation of the nerves) extends into the fourth year. These varying rates of growth have vital implications not only to the child's nutritional requirements at such times but also to any mechanical factors that hinder the developing nervous system. For optimal growth and development, the brain and all the body parts need to develop in balance and harmony with each other.

Spinal development

Each one of us has our own unique working pattern, depending on our genes, birth and constitution. When we reach adulthood we have a dominant side of the body from which we tend to position ourselves and the body is often asymmetrical. The body is comfortable in this working pattern, so there might be a short leg on one side or a bend on the top of the spine. The body also continually adapts to the various stresses and strains of life, and these too will add to the variations in the basic working pattern. The baby's body, on the other hand, has not yet been influenced in these ways. A child's posture is important for growth and development; for example, as the head sits balanced on the neck and shoulders, the eyes and ears need to be level so that maximum information can be gleaned from the environment.

The type of posture adopted by the body largely depends on how the spinal curves develop. While in the uterus the baby is curled up, so there is only one C-shaped spinal curve, known as the primary curve. After birth, the baby gradually learns to hold up his head against the compressive forces of gravity. This helps the spinal curves to develop in the neck and lower back in the opposite direction to the original C. However, the presence of compression strains at certain areas of the body will influence the development of the spine and pelvis.

Although any deviation from the normal posture is mostly seen in the spine, it is also present in the head. For example, an oblique-shaped skull at birth creates an unequal pull on either side of the developing muscles of the neck and spine. The body grows into this asymmetry, associated with which will be a deviation of the pelvis and shoulders. This does not cause any symptoms in the infant, but the deviation increases with growth, and secondary compensatory changes in other structures are produced. These are usually not a problem until extra loads get added on to the body, when it may not cope well in response to some event in later life. As a result, a knock on the head or a fall on the bottom or even heavy dental work may create symptoms that are worse than the incident would appear to warrant.

While in the uterus or during labour, the baby's body is subject to compression and certain areas are more affected than others: the cranium, top of the neck and upper back are particularly vulnerable. As we saw in chapter five, it is not uncommon to find retained compression in other areas such as the middle of the back and pelvis, and the baby naturally finds a position of comfort for that part of the body. Take the example of strain within the pelvis. The development of the hips may be influenced by the alteration of the shape of the ball and socket joints. Equally, an altered relationship with the spine at the coccyx and sacrum can affect the structures and the nerves to the bladder and pelvic organs. In an older child, this may be the mechanical cause of bedwetting or constipation and later, in the teenage years, of painful periods. However, the osteopath can work to release the compression strains, balancing tension throughout the spine and its membranous network so that the growing body is not overly stressed.

Development and learning

The course of the brain's development is long and drawn-out. Most brain development occurs when the baby is in the uterus, and it continues at a declining rate post-natally. The forebrain and the brain stem, for example, have reached only 70 per cent of their mature values when the child is two years of age. A mechanical restriction to the growing brain limits the space available for growth and acts like any joint restriction elsewhere in the body, where the organ's nutrition is affected through altered blood supply and venous and lymphatic drainage mechanisms.

During the growing years, there are relatively short periods of time when the brain's growth spurts means that it is vulnerable to under-nutrition, mechanical or environmental factors. At these times, the brain seizes on whatever stimulus is available for the development of a particular aspect of learning. If the right kind of stimulus is not there, an unsuitable pattern is learnt; the need for both visual and auditory stimuli is essential at these times, especially after six months when the baby begins to move around more. If he can hear his mother he will feel secure in learning that she is not far away even when he can't see her. If the hearing stimulus is reduced then the developmental opportunity for speech is impeded. Fortunately, the brain is relatively plastic for a short time, during which problems can be addressed, as demonstrated in George's case below.

The complex processes of learning and development are based on motion and activity. A new baby arrives with motion reflexes – such as suckling – and he learns about things by reaching for objects seen and then grasped in the hand. He responds to sounds that will eventually help him to formulate speech. So, as we all know, it is vital that the growing child can see, hear and move properly.

Sight

Occasionally, newborn babies have 'cross-eyes' or squints, which usually settle as the baby gets older and the eye muscles become stronger. One of the effects of retained cranial moulding is on the eyes. Each eye socket is composed of seven bones and any physical distortion within the cranium and face will affect the shape of the socket.

The eyeball is a fluid-filled fibrous structure whose shape can become changed in response to the compressive forces of the socket, so that the ability to focus is affected. The response to these forces can also create an unequal tension in the muscles controlling the eye movements, which results in an unequal pull of the eyeball. In addition, the nerves that supply the different muscle sets are also subject to cranial distortion and compression, and this too affects the ability to see. As the child gets older, undue tension in the muscles and the shape of the eyeball means that he may not be able to see letters very well or the lines jump. He may also have difficulty in copying from the chalkboard and be prone to headaches when reading. It is vital to establish and correct the optical reasons for eye problems. Cranial distortion and its effects on both the eyeball and its socket are easier to correct soon after the baby is born, but the body's capacity to correct itself, even in latter years, is surprising and rewarding.

Hearing

GEORGE'S DIFFICULTIES

George's mother was worried. At the age of five he was a handful, and he was not yet speaking properly. He often caught colds and had already taken four courses of antibiotics for ear infections. His latest hearing test was poor and grommets were being considered.

George's birth had been difficult. The labour had been over 20 hours and he was born with forceps. When I examined him I especially felt the birth strain at the temporal bones in the cranial base, where the membranes attached to these bones were tight and distorted. This state of affairs was affecting George's eardrums and he was suffering with congestive deafness or 'glue ear', which probably felt as if he were wearing cotton wool. Because he could not hear words properly, his speech was affected, and he naturally became frustrated and unruly.

The structures of the ears are contained in the temporal bones. These bones are originally composed of three parts and in a difficult birth have the capacity to slightly shift in relation to each other (just like the occipital bone) and its neighbouring bones. As George grew, the distorted strain pattern became ingrained, restricting movement and interfering with the drainage of the middle ear. Normally, the ear drains into the back of the throat via the eustachian tube, and the movements of the cranial bones augment this. By itself, restricted motion of the temporal bone is not a problem. Although the function of the tube is compromised, it is still adequate – until there is an added load, such as a cold. An infection or even a toxic reaction to a routine immunization causes the tonsils and adenoids to become enlarged. These lymphatic tissues lie near the eustachian tube and so partially block the drainage from the ear. Pressure then builds up behind it, which can be painful and in excess may cause the eardrum to burst. Such problems are often accompanied by poor mechanics of the neck so that the lymph channels here also become congested. As the ear cannot drain properly, it becomes a breeding ground for reinfection. Eventually, a sticky residue remains and the 'glue ear' can cause reduced hearing. Glue ear is now often treated by the use of grommets, which can provide an effective remission, but healing leaves a scar on the eardrum which may affect hearing in later life.

It was also noted that George opened his bowels only every other day, which added to the generally poor elimination of substances within the body.

George's treatment began by my correcting the cranial mechanics, the relationships of the temporal bones and their attached membranes. The lymphatic and venous drainage from the head and the neck was improved, and the ears began to clear. When his diet was changed to include more fruit and vegetables and I did some work on the gut as well as the spinal and pelvic areas, George began to open his bowels more regularly. This also reduced the build-up of catarrh. But, in the long run, he needed help with his immune function to fight off infections. After a few months, George's hearing began to improve in spite of his getting colds. As he began to hear words more clearly, his speech naturally got better. The temporal lobes, which are crucial to the understanding of speech, lie in the proximity of the temporal bones, and now had more space within which to function. George was at last getting the right auditory input and this stimulated the function of the speech centres. He could finally hear what people were saying, and answer without feeling frustrated.

Infections

Infections in a child are a natural process to enable the immune system to develop antibodies in the battle against the bug. But some children do tend to be more vulnerable to reinfections. Often there is a history of a difficult birth or the mother had some distress during the pregnancy. In these circumstances the overall vitality and immune function of the growing child is likely to be affected. Either there may be a tendency towards allergies and intolerances, or the ability to fight off infections is impaired. When an infection seems rather prolonged, it is often because the body has a mechanical problem with clearing away the debris.

WALTER AND HIS TROUBLES

Walter was a two-year-old Down's syndrome baby and had been referred by his GP for help with recurrent colds and coughs. Down's syndrome occurs because of a chromosomal abnormality that affects the growth of the foetus. The nervous system is immature and the skeleton is also affected. The muscles are flabby, and the growth of the facial bones and the ends of the limbs tends to be slow, contributing to typical features. Learning difficulties, mild or severe, are also associated with Down's children. The critical stages in the development are affected during prenatal growth, yet there is more marked retardation after the birth. The growth deficiency causes a shortening of the cranial base and the bones of the face, which affects not only the developing central nervous system but also the space of the airways. In turn, this affects breathing and the ability of the upper respiratory tract to drain mucus, which was Walter's problem.

Sinuses are air cavities that are formed in the cranial bones. The bones of the face on either side of the nose and in the forehead are responsible for filtering the air we breathe and also for the drainage of the mucous membranes of the head and face. Their shape is genetically predisposed, but is also influenced by unresolved birth compression through the middle of the face. However, because of Down's syndrome, the bones forming Walter's sinuses were so small as to be almost absent.

When movement between the bones of the cranium is limited, it inhibits the drainage mechanisms of the mucous membranes that line them. Excess mucus is not cleared away, and the blocked nose becomes habitual. After a while, poor drainage sets up an environment that is vulnerable to infection, especially if a child is a mouth breather. The mucous membranes that line the sinuses and the upper respiratory tract – the middle ear, mastoid and throat – are continuous. Inhaled irritants such as house dust or pollen can stimulate excessive secretion of mucus through the reaction of the sympathetic ganglia lying at the top of the cheekbones. This causes irritation of the nose's mucous membranes and is a contributing cause of sinusitis, asthma and recurrent middle ear infections. So when the osteopath treats, she not only deals with the problem area but also helps to improve the overall immune function.

With treatment aimed at maintaining the drainage mechanisms, Walter's health began to improve. His whole body was worked on, with special emphasis on creating better function through the chest, head and face. With fewer colds, he could breathe more easily so more oxygen became available for his developing nervous system. In addition, the work on the cranium meant more space was available for the brain and spinal cord and so the conditions for Walter's growth and development were optimized.

Asthma

Asthma occurs when there is an inflammation and narrowing of the airways, which makes it difficult to breathe. It is triggered by various factors such as house dust, animal dander, cigarette or traffic fumes, influenza, dairy products or nuts, and thick mucus is produced. Symptoms usually start with a long-lasting cough, which is worse at night, often after exercise or where there is anxiety. There is shortness of breath and the chest feels tight and wheezy. The extent of symptoms is variable, ranging from a distressing cough to tremendous difficulty in breathing, which requires hospitalization. Although asthma is increasing, there is little understanding of the relationship of the body structure to the function of the lungs. Medication is essential in cases of severe asthma, but improving the mechanics of the body can greatly enhance the breathing mechanics as well as the ability to cope with factors which trigger an attack. Also, because osteopaths work so much on the chest to improve the function of the overall body, most chest afflictions tend to respond well.

Medications usually consist of 'relievers' taken to relax the muscles of the airways so they can open. Such medications act in a similar manner to adrenaline, which the body naturally produces to get ready for action and they can contribute to over-activity in children. They are generally taken in conjunction with 'preventers', which treat inflammation of the airways to stop symptoms from appearing when exposed to triggers.

DAVID'S ASTHMA

David was a lively five-year-old. He was suffering from asthma, which was kept under control by the use of inhalers. But his mother said that there were times when he was so active that he could not be calmed down. He was born suddenly at 34 weeks of pregnancy and required ventilation to help him breathe.

When I examined David, I noticed there was a sense of tightness throughout the body, but more so around the chest. The muscles of the neck and rib cage were working too hard because of poor excursion of the ribs, the spinal joints, and the diaphragm and other muscles of breathing. In addition, the fascias that envelop the lungs and the throat felt tight and inelastic, which further limited lung function. From feeling the cranium, it was evident that the normal processes of suckling or crying had not completely resolved the effects of the birth strain. There was also a heavy and sluggish feel in the tissues, to which the medications probably contributed.

David's treatment was initially aimed at helping his chest and rib cage to expand fully. This would allow the soft tissues and fascias to give space for the motion of the lungs. But first the effects of birth strain and distress needed to be eased out of the body through releasing and balancing the cranial and spinal membranes right into the coccyx. This also helped the mechanisms of breathing, especially as the diaphragm was eased, so that with each breath the thorax began to work more efficiently. This work also improved the venous drainage, circulation and the flow of lymphatic fluid through the chest, which would help him to fight off infection.

David's asthma often came on when he got anxious or felt overwhelmed, which in turn disturbed the autonomic pathways to the lungs. These were balanced by relaxing the cranial and spinal areas connected with the hypothalamus and the autonomic nervous system. When the lymphatic drainage was improved, David's body became more efficient at metabolizing the medication. Over a few months this ameliorated the fluid quality and texture of his tissues, which became more elastic and supple. As a result he became less charged-up and needed less medication. David's mother now brings him as his prolonged cough comes on or when he is in contact with known triggers, in order to help prevent an attack.

Learning difficulties

A plethora of labels is used to describe these problems, depending on which brain activity is affected. Some of the common ones are attention deficit disorder, autism, hyperactivity, speech disorder, dyslexia, dyspraxia or minimal brain dysfunction. There are many factors – nutritional, genetic, environmental, social and psychological – which contribute to these problems. Often such children are intelligent, but unfortunately the capacity to express and develop that capability is hindered. In almost 80 per cent of cases there is a history of traumatic birth and associated problems with the framework and structural and functional relationships of the body.

WILLIAM'S SCHOOLDAYS

Twelve-year-old William seemed like a bright lad, but his school reports suggested otherwise. Although he enjoyed school and had friends, he found the lessons hard. He had difficulty in reading, spelling or understanding what was written. His ability to recall was poor and his writing was untidy and sprawling. He knew he could do better, but somehow could not express what was in his head.

Becky, his mother, had been poorly with nausea and vomiting through the first three months of the pregnancy and the labour had been awful. William had an odd-shaped head, indicating severe compression, and there had been a slight delay in taking his first breath. As a baby, he was very demanding, sleeping for only short periods of time. After weaning, he was a fussy eater and mealtimes were difficult. He potty-trained easily and reached his milestones at the right times and liked being on the move.

At the age of two William was standing behind the door as Becky pushed it open. He knocked his head and was inconsolable for the next few days. At the age of four, it was discovered that he couldn't see very well and needed glasses. At nursery school, he had not got on well with his teacher, who thought William was awkward. He was a fidget, going from one activity to the next within minutes; at times, he was disruptive, even in the playground. Although not good at ball games, he enjoyed athletics and riding his bicycle. When he went to high school he lagged behind his peers and his self-worth was shaken. As he entered his teens, William's diet consisted mainly of cereals, bread, pizza, crisps, chocolates and fizzy drinks, having fruit only if it was cut for him.

William's difficulties were due to several things. He had dyslexia, which is an inability to read, spell or write words, despite the ability to see and recognize letters. He also had mild dyspraxia, which is difficulty with balance and with the co-ordination of muscles. Fine motor skills, such as those needed for the hand control required to write, were hard for him, as were the gross motor skills needed for catching a ball. However, most learning difficulties are not as clear-cut as their labels would suggest and there is interplay of several factors.

A difficult birth had left William with residual compression strain throughout the body but especially in the cranium. This would have meant he was very uncomfortable, probably with a persistent headache. As he grew, William avoided the physical discomfort felt in his body by constantly being on the move, so he didn't really learn to concentrate for periods of time. In addition, the poor eyesight so early on and difficulty sleeping had made him irritable and aggravated the poor concentration. The knock to William's head compounded his problems coping with distortions persisting from birth. After the age of seven, as the sutures of the skull became fully developed, William's nervous system found it harder to accommodate growth and added stress loads. Once at senior school, William was expected to be still and focus on one task for extended periods of time and this was a huge effort. He could not keep up and was left very tired, frustrated and irritable. Just as William's tissues felt tight and unable to express their inherent motion fully, so too he had difficulty expressing his personality.

William's treatment regime needed several approaches. His osteopathic treatment was geared to removing the musculoskeletal restrictions brought about at birth and the trauma of the bang to his head. Easing the cranial distortions helped to remove the restrictions to the brain and eyes and the nervous system. The different brain parts could then integrate better and develop a new pattern of function. Because William did not eat balanced meals, he may have lacked essential nutrients required at the vulnerable periods of growth. So his parents were advised on a nutritional regime that favoured brain nourishment.

Underlying William's problems were some emotional difficulties. Initially, an unsympathetic nursery teacher left him feeling that school experiences would be unhappy – and now the high expectations, which he struggled to meet, left him feeling depressed. William was given one-to-one tuition and, although he found academic subjects difficult to grasp, he was good at art where his imagination could take over. He was encouraged to express himself through this and over time his artwork took on a freer flowing quality, having previously been more cramped and restricted, just like his body.

William was treated intensively for the first two months and after that he was seen once a month. A year later, his proud father presented William's school report which showed an immense improvement all round, and he even developed a liking for science subjects.

Developmental delay and brain damage

Many developmental problems occur because of impaired functional processes of the brain. In these cases, the brain is not starved of oxygen, but it works in a disturbed manner. Its functional ability can also be modified by many factors, such as disturbed biochemistry, the position of the head on the neck, muscular pulls and fascial drags from the base of the skull, as well as misalignments of the cranial bones and their attached membranes. But, by removing the mechanical impediments to brain motion, such as those found within the cranium, neck and the sacrum, the neurological function can be greatly enhanced. For example, the area that takes a large brunt of the compression forces at birth is the cranial base at the back of the head. The cerebellum, which lies at the back of the brain in the region of the occipital bone, grows rapidly and achieves adult values by two years of age. So the removal of any mechanical compression of birth in this area, preferably before the age of two, will mean the functions of the cerebellum, such as co-ordination of movements, are much improved.

Damaged brain cells are another cause of neurological dysfunction. The osteopath feels such damage as a sense of heaviness within the brain, which also feels small. This kind of damage occurs if there has been a lack of oxygen so that some cells die, and it can also happen if there is a bleed into the brain tissues or in a particularly difficult birth when the brain swells. While the damaged cells cannot be repaired, it is possible to enhance the function of other cells of the brain. This helps to improve the overall function of the central nervous system, especially if a baby is treated soon after birth. By removing bony and membranous restrictions to the motions of the central nervous system, encouraging the blood flow and reducing venous congestion within the cranium, the osteopath can help to develop the child's potential, albeit within the limits of the degree of brain damage.

CHARLIE'S TALKING

Charlie's mother cautioned me to keep my distance – he was spitting again and using anything moving as a target. At the grand age of five Charlie was an old patient of the practice, attending since he was eight months old. At birth, he was a floppy, blue baby who had suffered from a lack of oxygen to the brain (anoxia). Although the pregnancy had been fine, Charlie got very distressed during birth, emptying his bowels before being born. He needed resuscitation but the damage to the brain left him with slow growth and development and he was now confined to a wheelchair. When the labour is so difficult as to cause anoxia, it also causes trauma to the baby so there is excessive cranial moulding with accompanying compression within the body tissues. Charlie could not control his movements and he needed help with everything.

Although osteopathy could not help the already damaged brain cells, much could be done to release the shock and distress from his system. This helped to release the moulding pressures of labour and the resultant strains within the tissues so that his body could start cranking into action. Because Charlie was seen early, much could be done to help with the patterning of new brain cells as they were still developing. As the restrictions within the cranium were released, the inherent motion within the cerebrospinal fluid and the brain tissues could be expressed more freely. This meant that although the functions of Charlie's body would never be normal, they would make an attempt. He had a lot of treatment so that his nervous system could have the best chance to develop within its obvious limitations. Charlie eventually began to spit when his speech and vocal areas were stimulated – this was a new activity for him, where he had learned to use his tongue in a novel attempt to talk.

For children like Charlie, the simplest things are extremely difficult and therefore any small change is a big event. By working on the structure of the body, much can be done to help those small changes along and give the body the opportunity to function slightly differently. Although life can never be normal, as we perceive it, even the tiniest thing is enough to alter the quality of life – Charlie's spitting was an accomplishment for him.

The effect of correcting any disturbances, large and small, can greatly enhance the growing child's potential. And when structural dysfunction from birth trauma is corrected early, all the body's functions have the maximum chance to develop.

Chapter seven

Life changes

No explorer can accurately forecast what he may encounter along the way, what the time involvement may be, or the precise destination. This is as true of anatomical-physiological exploration as it is of archeological, oceanographic or others.

Adah Strand Sutherland

EMILY'S TRANSFORMATION

'Now don't run late, you've got Emily coming in at eleven o' clock and you know what a dragon she can be!' advised my receptionist, who dreaded her visits. Emily was an aggressive, high-powered businesswoman who was extremely focused, usually on her needs. Driven mostly by her adrenals, she came across as hard and uncompromising. Although her prime concern was an injury to the knee caused by a skiing accident, she also had lower back problems. In the background was a history of irregular menstrual cycles, her periods occurring once every three to four months. The knee and lower back only took a few sessions to clear, but the problems of the sacrum and pelvis were more stubborn. In addition, there was an underlying imbalance of the autonomic nervous system, extending right from the hormonal glands in the cranium to the adrenal glands in the back.

Emily was therefore seen every six weeks for the next six months. During one such appointment, the receptionist declared what a pleasant, nice lady Emily was and hadn't she changed? Although she still had an odd menstrual cycle, her body had become less charged up as it had begun to function more efficiently, and this was reflected in a new calmer self. She could now embrace the world and interact with it from a more relaxed perspective, so much so that a year later she was diligently practising yoga. She has now given up her business and teaches yoga.

Hormones and the body

When we think about life changes, we generally think about the physical transformation of the body. We link these changes with the major hormonal influences at puberty, childbirth and menopause, the significant physical changes associated with age. Events such as disease or trauma, however, also modify the body's normal physiological processes and we cannot continue our normal lifestyle. By the same token, as the body function improves, the desire to change our lifestyle can become stronger. As their body is released of its stresses and strains, people often gain the courage and self-confidence to make major changes in their lives. Those people who are naturally driven in character, like Emily, while remaining driven may attain the ability to control it.

The physical body is the instrument through which we express our inner self. We have an idea, a thought about what we want to do and how we want to do it, and through the body we can process that idea to make it our reality. But when the body is not working well there is a limit to what we can achieve. Hormones maintain the body's smooth running and its rhythms, and these vary in levels over the day, night, weeks, months, even years. Although there may not be a major hormonal problem, subtle shifts within the endocrine balance are registered by equally subtle changes within the body. So when you visit the osteopath she may ask what seem to be irrelevant questions in relation to your pain or discomfort. You might be asked if you are prone to tiredness and if so at what times of the day, if you are subject to recurrent colds, or coldness in the hands and/or feet, moodiness at certain times of the day and/or month, if you have suffered from sudden weight loss/gain. These give an indication of how the body is working hormonally in relation to its whole function.

Hormones are chemicals released into the bloodstream by the endocrine glands. Because blood permeates every single cell and organ of the body, all the cells are affected. As a result, too much or too little hormone has far-reaching consequences. So a lack of certain hormones can make the muscles more susceptible to spasm and therefore pain. Cramps, aching in the legs and feet or general stiffness may be related to the parathyroid hormone, which is responsible for the balance of calcium in the body. In children, an insufficiency of growth hormone can be one of the reasons for slow growth (along with factors relating to poor nutrition, emotional starvation or stress).

Osteopaths believe that motion is essential to efficient body function, and the endocrine glands are no exception. Two glands present in the brain itself, the pituitary and the pineal, are important, particularly the former – the 'king-pin' of all hormonal glands.

The pineal is a small gland found towards the front of the brain and seems to affect the daily and seasonal cycles of the body. It is partly responsible for the seasonal affective disorder (SAD syndrome) where altered production of melatonin during the winter months leads to depressive states. In Eastern philosophy the pineal gland is considered to be the seat of intuitive knowledge and some paranormal attributes such as telepathic communication. We do not yet fully understand all the functions of this gland but it influences the regulation of sleep, mood, puberty and ovarian cycles.

The pituitary gland is the most complex of all hormonal glands and influences all the other endocrine glands. It is divided into two parts. The front secretes nourishment hormones that are important in regulating the growth and activity of both the body as a whole and of other endocrine glands. The back part is important in the production of urine and it also releases hormones that cause rhythmic contractions during birth. The pituitary sits above the roof of the mouth and nasal cavity, where it is responsive to motion in the cranium and related structures. The pituitary gland connects to the hypothalamus, and both this and the pineal gland have stalks, which are like tubes that open into the interconnecting fluid compartments or ventricles of the brain. This means that with each fluctuating motion of the CSF and alternating motion of the brain, whose membranes are attached to the movable cranial bones and sacrum, there is an equally minute but significant motion of these glands. Using the motion of primary respiration therefore enables the osteopath to help balance the endocrine function.

Change and growth

There is much written about the influence of the mind on the body (some books are noted in the reading list on pages 155–56). It is well known that some illnesses are more common among those with certain personality traits; allergies, for example, are often identified as being the somatic response of a sensitive person who does not always externalize his feelings. Just as the mind can influence how the body reacts, functional changes within the body also affect how we feel about ourselves. When we do not feel well or are in pain, it is not easy to make changes, and even making simple decisions can be quite difficult. If the body feels sluggish, stiff and slow, the mind may reflect this. But as the body function recovers we feel recharged and the personality becomes stronger.

With the growing popularity of mind-body medicine, more people are taking responsibility for their spiritual and physical wellbeing. Just as there are physical changes in the body related to age, extensive research in the field of ageing by Levinson and others seems to show that psychological change also occurs according to a schedule of chronological phases. These are the early adult phase, the adult phase, mid-life transition and the middle adult years. All of these are times when the body is rapidly changing. Moody and Carrol in their book *The Five Stages of the Soul* indicate that there are specific stages of spiritual awakening that we go through as we age. For many people there is the 'mid-life crisis' which is related to the search for inner purpose, and fulfilment is achieved once the path to spiritual wholeness has been found. Associated with these transitions are physical changes occurring within the body. The body will often groan with aches and pains as the tissues process this inner work. As the shifts are made within, they are experienced in the body; having osteopathy to retune the body can help to make such a transition more harmonious.

For some people, certain events will alter their path in life and these can create havoc in the body function although there might not be any overt disease. Emotional trauma or shock are such events. Witnessing an accident or

Figure 14 THE MAJOR HORMONAL GLANDS OF THE BODY

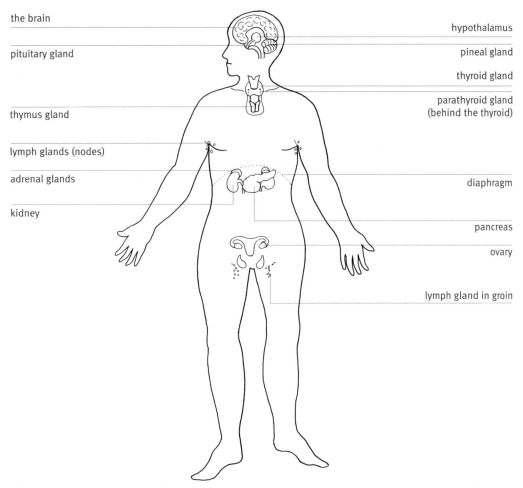

the brain

pituitary gland

thymus gland

lymph glands (nodes)

adrenal glands

kidney

hypothalamus

pineal gland

thyroid gland

parathyroid gland
(behind the thyroid)

diaphragm

pancreas

ovary

lymph gland in groin

Pituitary gland: found at the base of the brain and attached by a stalk to the hypothalamus; has two lobes and orchestrates the hormonal structures of the body, secreting many different hormones. Controls functions including the thyroid gland, sex hormones, female hormonal cycles and ovulation, growth, water content of the body, and steroid production by adrenal glands.

Hypothalamus: integrates autonomic mechanisms, endocrine (hormonal) activity and other metabolic body functions such as sleep, temperature regulation, food intake and onset of puberty.

Pineal gland; implicated in regulation of sleep, mood, puberty and ovarian cycles.

Thyroid gland: has two lobes. Regulates metabolic rates of the body (metabolism is the sum of all physical and chemical processes and energy release required for the maintenance of life) and temperature.

Parathyroid gland: behind the thyroid gland. Regulates calcium and phosphorus metabolism.

Lymph glands and thymus gland: produce lymphocytes associated with immune function.

Adrenal glands: lie on top of each kidney. Respond to physical and psychological stress.

Pancreas: lies behind the stomach. Secretes the hormone insulin, which regulates blood sugar levels of the body, as well as enzymes needed for digestion of protein.

Ovary: two glands in the female, which produce eggs during the monthly cycle.

hearing tragic news stirs up excess energy with nowhere to go, overloading the system with emotional strain patterns. When this excess energy is allowed to dissipate by restoring the rhythmic motion throughout its tissues, the body will calm down, and greater clarity of thought often follows.

Although each of us is a complete whole unit of function, our survival depends on our being part of larger units, part of a group – the family unit, the people we work with, the community in which we live. These people form our environment and so when something happens to them not only are we affected but those dependent on us will also be affected by our reactions. An African witchdoctor was asked to heal some patients who had been psychologically traumatized. As is usual in Western practice, he was ushered into a room, for a one-to-one meeting with his patient. To this he exclaimed, 'Where is the village – I can't work without the village!' For this man, the villagers' goodwill for the person played a large part in the healing process. This is also important from an osteopathic point of view when treating families, since altered dynamics may interfere with a harmonious function of the family unit.

TOBY'S AGGRESSION

Glenda had originally brought little Toby because of very mild cerebral palsy. He had been a pleasure to treat and had responded very well until two months ago. Recently he had become aggressive, quite disobedient and verging on the hyperactive. On feeling his tissues, I thought that Toby seemed fine in himself, except that his psychic point of orientation was lodged in his mother, rather than in the middle of his own body. When feeling Glenda's shoulders, the excessive tension here indicated an underlying problem. She had been looking after her mother who had had a serious stroke, since when she had become withdrawn and Glenda was unable to communicate with her on even the most essential levels. This preyed on Glenda's mind and she felt helpless in not knowing how to cater to her mother's needs. The whole family revolved around Glenda and she ordinarily kept the dynamics well balanced. However, as she became preoccupied with her mother, Toby, who had his own difficulties and needed extra care, just could not function from his own centre. That session, Glenda was treated instead of Toby, to calm her down and allow her body to become a place of relative stillness. As a result, Toby regained his centre and the family equilibrium came to a better state of balance.

Eventually this life's journey will come to a close. But although the physical functions of the body deteriorate, the person and the physical body can still be supported through the final stages. Sarah's life changed dramatically after her car accident, which was described on page 77. As we saw, she had not suffered any breakage of bones and made some recovery as far as injuries to her neck and back were concerned. However, she had previously suffered with multiple health problems and her mother had died of breast cancer. This final trauma of the car accident had, over a period of time, unfortunately tipped the balance for her and she also succumbed to breast cancer. With drug therapy, she went into remission and continued to work for a while, but a year later the cancer spread. As with Margaret, whose final illness was described at the beginning of the book, osteopathy contributed towards keeping her comfortable, easing the stresses and strains out of her tissues, reducing the pain and helping her to feel a quality of stillness within. Both Sarah and Margaret were helped to come to terms with their final passage towards death.

GRACE'S LAST ILLNESS

Grace was 72 years old and ill. She had had several operations on various joints for her rheumatoid arthritis but was brought into the practice because she easily got very breathless. She had originally suffered with a persistent dry cough which a later chest scan revealed to be a malignant tumour sitting behind the heart. And now it had spread – but Amanda, her daughter, indicated to me that Grace had chosen not to know about its progress, although she knew that these were her final months. Amanda was concerned about her mother's comfort and fear of what lay beyond.

Grace could not lie flat as she would instantly dissolve into a fit of coughing. As she lay, half inclined, my hands sensed a lot of business in the tissues. They were preoccupied with dealing with the medication, the stress of making the journey out to my practice, with the feeling that she was inconveniencing her family and a lot else besides. Gradually as her compensatory mechanisms began to be put aside, a sense of calm emerged. As the tissues gradually relaxed, the whole body began to express the motions of primary respiration as a single unit – there was no sense of mind, body and psyche being separate. I could do no more for her in this session, as the tissues had had enough. The next time I saw Grace she remarked that the breathlessness and the cough were much better, and as an aside Amanda said how peaceful Grace had become. This session I felt a deep sense of inertia, mainly in the lungs. I sat with this for what seemed a long time, and then it seemed to melt and the whole body softened.

Four weeks later, Grace had become very ill; she was retaining fluid in her abdomen and asked to be treated in order to feel calm. On this occasion, as the treatment came to an end Grace fell asleep; she felt good, the rhythm felt very strong and cohesive within the whole body, and this seemed to permeate the whole room. She died four days later, at peace with herself and with permission to go from her loved ones.

Dr Still, the father of osteopathy, called the body the 'second placenta', as a way of expressing that some unknown birth takes place at the time of death. An osteopath works with the innate healing forces to help relieve the mind of clutter and allow fear to melt so that the natural and orderly process of death can come to pass with ease. Amanda, who had been pregnant during her mother's illness, later recalled that when her granddaughter was two weeks old Grace had remarked, 'I can go now.'

Chapter eight

How the body responds to treatment

The body of man is God's drug store and has in it all the liquids, drugs, lubricating oils, opiates, acids and antacids and every sort of drug that the wisdom of God thought necessary for human happiness and health.

Dr Andrew Taylor Still

The effects of the light touch method of osteopathy in the cranial field are profound and yet to the person watching, or indeed receiving, treatment it appears that the osteopath is merely sitting there, holding the head, pelvis or some other part of the body. The effects of the treatment are varied and while some of these are felt during the session, other responses may occur a day or so later; sometimes even a week later. Some people can relate quite specifically how their body functioning has changed, others just know that they feel different.

During the treatment, the osteopath is meeting the needs of the body and encouraging the patient's body to make the corrections, so that the tissues change their behavioural patterns and in the long run are not strained. More often than not, the experience of being treated is very pleasant and soothing. Occasionally people may experience odd sensations such as warmth or heat, others feel a sense of liquid energy and yet others see fabulous colours. Sometimes people may even register that the boundary of their physical body melts, leaving no sense of delineation between them and the room. Other people may feel nothing at all.

Patients quite commonly feel increased pain at the site of the offending problem. There is an awareness of being uncomfortable and this is usually followed by a need to stretch. The discomfort mostly lasts only as long as the consultation and usually at the end there is much relief (often to the surprise of the patient). Occasionally when there has been a previous trauma and the resultant stresses and strain within the tissues are released, the patient may feel an intense pain at the site of the problem. This pain is from the tissue memory of the old trauma and usually only lasts briefly within the treatment session. As the memory is released, the osteopath feels a turbulent motion of the tissues as they dissipate the 'pent-up' energy, which is often released as heat, twitching or shaking of part or the whole body. Occasionally when nerves are released the accompanying sensation may be one of burning, which can be unnerving and rather uncomfortable. It may only be momentary or it can last a while, until the residual inflammation subsides. Old falls or accidents or injuries are often forgotten with the passage of time. As they are released from the tissues, however, it is not unusual for the patient to recall the course of events as they occurred. This may happen immediately or within a few days of treatment.

At times, a patient may feel uncomfortable or ache after the session – sometimes it can feel like having done five rounds with Mike Tyson! This usually comes on a few hours or a day later and may last about two to three days, occasionally even for a week. Rollin Becker describes this colourfully: '[patients] can actually feel worse because you have given orders to the tissues, the fascias, the connective tissues, which like to do the loudest screaming. You woke them up. An unhealthy tissue does not wake up and say, "Oh, joy, peace in the world!" It wakes up and says, "Who the hell told you to disturb me?" ' When part of the body has not been working properly strains can occur as the body compensates for the original injury. When motion is reinstated within these tissues there can be a sense of aching such as you might feel from a work-out after a period of inactivity. Fortunately, this usually only happens early on within the treatment programme. Thereafter, as the tissues get better function through them, they become less reactive and the symptoms simply melt away.

Often patients come to an osteopath having been advised that a condition will just run its natural course and finally ease away. This may well be the case, but usually there is a cost. It may be that the condition persists for a long time and the body may then have to resolve the condition by compensating for it elsewhere. These secondary effects may not be evident in the short term but become so years later, when further strains are taken into the body. Back pain, for example, may resolve by itself, depending on the cause, and patients are often advised to rest. But it is not always practical to take weeks upon weeks of total rest and neither does this actually resolve the problem. Equally, parents are often advised that colic is common during the first three months of life, after which it ceases. This screaming after feeding is awful for both mother and baby and there is often little need to wait this long – depending on the cause, babies are often made comfortable within one to three sessions. Similarly, when the older child complains of various aches and pains or allergies, parents are advised that the child will grow out of it. Although osteopathic treatment cannot stop the condition when it has already begun its course, its duration and often the intensity of discomfort can be greatly reduced. Treatment encourages the body to resolve any unwanted forces and correct its mechanics, so that the self-healing responses are not hindered and the health of the body is supported.

The effects of osteopathy are to improve the body's physiology. This means that as the various tissues of the body – the joints, muscles and internal organs – are activated, their function improves. A major effect is on the nervous system, especially the autonomic component, so that the digestion and metabolism of food is improved. As a result, during treatment the stomach often rumbles and babies may want to feed.

Because osteopathy improves the physiology of the body, when there is an infection, such as a cold brewing, the symptoms may get worse straight after treatment. This is because the immune system is mobilized into action and the treatment can act as a catalyst to the normal reactions. Where a cold would normally last for a week to ten days, its course will be much shorter and occasionally slightly more intense. The circulation, lymphatic and drainage mechanisms have been improved and so the runny nose or coughing increases temporarily to clear the wasted debris from the body. This can sometimes temporarily aggravate a toxic condition such as eczema. When an infection is caught early enough it can be nipped in the bud; if not, then it will occur but run a much shorter course. Due to improved physiology, any remedies or medicines taken are readily absorbed and utilized by the gut, and their transport is made more efficient because of improved blood circulation. They become more potent as a result and it is therefore advisable that the prescribing practitioner monitors medication carefully, as the dosages may need reducing. This is particularly so in patients with epilepsy or asthma, to prevent over-medication.

For the majority of patients, and especially children, receiving treatment is a very pleasant experience. People often fall asleep, or certainly reach a deep state of relaxation. It is not uncommon for some irritable babies who have never settled after birth to stay asleep for a day or so, waking only to feed. There are other less tangible after-effects of osteopathic treatment that are also due to improved body physiology. The subtle changes within the tissues may be due to the fluid dynamics affecting the autonomic and endocrine nervous systems as well as the emotional centres. Different people are affected in different ways but there are similarities. Quoted below are some typical sensations.

VANESSA'S EXPERIENCE

I find it very relaxing on the whole. At first I found it made my mind race. I had all sorts of jumbled thoughts and felt very much that something was in my space. I grappled to control my mind as I do when I attempt to meditate. When I did finally calm my thoughts I went into deep relaxation. With each session my body and mind feel more balanced and I see my third eye each time. It appears in a sea of indigo/violet with a white eye-shape in the middle of my forehead: generally in meditation it takes an hour and a half of concentration for this to happen. After the treatment I feel very light and relaxed.

KATE'S EXPERIENCE

During treatment, almost always, a soft violet light spreads across my inner eyes. If I am lucky, this colour creeps right across my vision until it envelops my complete field of sight. If I am not so lucky, the violet light only partially appears and comes and goes.

I often have 'dreams', which include but are not restricted to a sensation of floating in space. This sensation has been enhanced on occasion by a very definite feeling of resting on air which is 'lapping' (as in lapping water). Throughout these dreams I feel completely safe, comfortable and surrounded by a loving unseen presence.

Often I experience a tingling sensation in hands and feet and almost physically feel the energy coursing through my limbs. Occasionally in the early days I would feel an unidentified emotion, gently moving from deep within me to the surface. Although unidentified in that I was not aware of the source or cause of this emotion, I did know that it was an emotion of sadness, and its cause was not important. What was important was that it was emerging and being released from me in such a gentle way, often accompanied by a few quiet tears.

After treatment I always have an enormous feeling of peace, inner calm and integration – the closest I have ever come to an understanding of serenity. A feeling of being with humanity but not part of it; almost as though I were wrapped in a cocoon of quiet and warmth.

Osteopathic treatment using primary respiration allows the body to make a shift in function at very deep levels of being. Depending on circumstances, we normally work in a state of compensation, where the different parts of the body are busy dealing with different things. In the city our body is revved up for dealing with the fumes, with the aggressive nature of people wanting to be somewhere five minutes ago, with digesting food we have bolted down for breakfast, with knowing that we won't be able to meet our personal or work schedule. All this requires compensatory mechanisms.

As the patient lies on the couch, the body is allowed to return to a level playing field, so that it becomes sufficiently balanced to reveal the actual problem. This may feel like you do when just returning from a holiday or spending the night under the stars. Patients do often seem to fall asleep, and it may be that the treatment brings about an altered state of consciousness, which allows the mechanisms of the nervous system an opportunity for processing autonomic and other physiological changes. These profound changes can occur because the inherent patterns of health are supported once the background 'noise' is reduced. As old working patterns of strain shift, the essential life force, or Breath of Life, can work in better functional patterns for the body. The patient occasionally experiences these new patterns through the release of light, heat and feelings of inner calm. But patients will not always have the same experiences in every session: as the body improves in its function and the tissues work more efficiently, treatment can be given as a preventive measure. The occasional tune-up helps the body to recover and regenerate quickly in response to the normal stresses and strains of daily life.

When it is suspected that the patient will ache after the treatment or has experienced any of the more marked sensations described above, they are usually advised to take some time to sit quietly and have a drink of water before venturing back out into the busy world. Because the body is working differently after treatment, the perception of the world is also that much altered and a few minutes of preparation may be needed.

Chapter nine

Maintaining wellness

And after all our explorations, we have to decide that man is triune when complete. First the material body, second the spiritual being, third a being of mind which is far superior to all vital motions and material forms, whose duty is to wisely manage this great engine of life.

Dr Andrew Taylor Still

Osteopathy in the cranial field is a method of manipulative medicine that works with primary respiration and the inherent motions of the body. These are seen by osteopaths to be the physical manifestation of the Breath of Life or the life force. While it is difficult to treat yourself with this method, anything that augments vitality and the expression of the life force will complement the work.

Although osteopathy works well with other methods of medicine, it is a method of healing in its own right. It is both complementary to all forms of medicine and yet also alternative; it supports all forms of medicine and yet is independent of all. Where there is debility from stroke or surgical intervention, it complements physiotherapy and occupational therapy. Where there is poor vitality osteopathy will support and speed up the process of herbs, medications, homeopathy, acupuncture and supplements of nutritional therapy.

One of the objectives of the osteopath is to ensure your comfort and trust during treatment. When these are achieved, there is less tension throughout the mind and body, and the work can take place more quickly. In order to help with this, I often suggest to the patient that he imagines himself in a place where he feels safe, relaxed and happy. It might be woodland, a beach, or a happy memory. Some patients use previously learned methods of relaxation or self-hypnosis techniques. Because your body dictates the treatment the osteopath will recognize from the behaviour of the tissues when to use, not use, or finish with a given procedure. So although the relaxation methods are not essential (nor is it a prerequisite to have faith in the process, which will happen anyway), I find they make it easier for the osteopath to work with the body.

Lifestyle

We all know that a day regularly balanced with both work and play is nourishing to the mind and body, even though it often seems hard to achieve when you are racing around getting your job done and looking after the kids. Although time management and discipline are needed if you are going to create this balance, you can help yourself by introducing some flexibility to a routine. If you have had a large supper with friends today, then you can re-establish balance by having a salad for lunch tomorrow. If you have had a long, draining day at work, it makes sense to go to bed early and not punish yourself further by going to the gym. You can make up the exercise tomorrow. Exercise needs to be regular, but does not have to be daily. Forty minutes three times a week should be enough, so long as you can also incorporate some daily walking into your time-management plan. Creative relaxation, hobbies such as music, seeing friends and having fun are essential aspects of looking after yourself. Sometimes we need to look at our values and beliefs to work out why we do what we do. It is important to include practices such as meditation or silence in your day, preferably at the same time and place each day. Work that you enjoy, preferably for which you have a talent, which stirs up some passion and challenges you constructively, will also help you to achieve the right kind of balance in life.

The food connection

The body needs fuel to maintain its structure. Taking in the right proportions of carbohydrates, fats, proteins, minerals and vitamins and fluids is essential in the production of energy, heat and growth and repair of the tissues.

In the West we tend to worry about being overweight, and tiredness is a common complaint. This has much to do with taking in food that offers little nourishment. Processed food may be tasty, but it can be lacking in terms of vitamins, minerals and essential fatty acids needed for the various physiological processes. These are vital for growing children, in particular, so it is unfortunate that they are often rewarded with fatty foods such as sweets, crisps or fizzy drinks, rather than fruit. Food not only carries energy, measured in terms of calories, but it also carries the same vital life force that is present in all living things. In some way, this affects the ability of the food substance to impart that energy; a packet of crisps or a bar of chocolate tastes lovely, but will not satisfy the body in the same way as a bunch of grapes.

Breakfast is the most essential meal of the day, since we are breaking a six to eight hours fast. There is a tendency either to miss it out completely or to have breakfast or lunch meetings so that we rarely concentrate on what is being eaten, let alone bother to chew it properly. When we consider that most traditional cultures have rituals around food, surely a society with a strong work ethic needs to allow half an hour or so for lunch? After all, this is the very food that will give us energy to live our busy lives, and it deserves respect. When there is no consideration given to the content or combination of the meal and it is eaten in a hurry, is it any wonder that we suffer with so many irritable bowel type symptoms?

Food intolerances and allergies seem to have increased markedly over the last thirty years and asthma now affects one in seven children in the UK. One contributory factor may be to do with modern methods of farming, including genetic engineering of crops, and food processing using additives, preservatives and colouring. Our digestive system has not yet evolved sufficiently to keep pace with these new developments. Then there are the effects of stress and anxiety: apart from its digestive function, the gut also connects us to our emotions. Sayings like 'gut feeling' or 'churning in the stomach' express this connection aptly. All too often anxiety is related to loose bowels or constipation. Most oriental self-defence systems such as karate use the solar plexus as a focus for 'grounding' or 'centring' oneself before a fight. It is regarded as the centre for personal power and this is not surprising when we consider that the developing foetus gains nutrition and energy from the umbilical cord.

There is much written about good nutrition and the interactions of various diets on different afflictions. There will always be different ideas about food and its effects on the body. But the important thing is that food should be as close as possible to its natural state and include plenty of variety.

Tips

• Never let the fridge go empty – that is when there is a tendency to binge on the bread, biscuits, crisps or anything else that is immediately available. Have vegetables, such as carrots, cauliflower, celery or mange-tout peas around, as they are easily nibbled and nourishing.
• Get a juicer. Juicing is essential for children who are fussy eaters, for busy people, and for those who have digestive difficulties, or are poorly or lacking in appetite. Juice can readily be made from a variety of fruits and vegetables. Carrots make a good base and mix with most substances.
• Try to have breakfast. Prepare it the night before, if you cannot get up earlier. Mixed fruit and yoghurt, organic muesli with fruit juice or porridge in the winter make good wholesome breakfasts. Again, variety is the key. Try to have the last meal about three hours before going to bed. If this is not possible, keep the last meal light.
• You should usually try to have some raw food with each meal. But don't do this if your bowels are going through an irritable phase, when you need to avoid roughage. You don't want to irritate them any further. At such a time, boiled rice, soups or broths are nourishing and easily digestible. Reintroduce the roughage once the acute phase is over and you have more energy to digest it.
• Drink plenty of water. An adult should take at least a litre daily.

The breath connection

The breath forms the universal and physiological connection. It is a powerful tool that integrates the different dimensions of our being (the unconscious with the conscious, the emotional and the spiritual with the physical) into a functional whole. The breath's significance extends from the requirement of oxygen for the biochemical processes of the internal organs to the subtle interplay of energy flow and its interactions with the mind.

Breathing begins with birth, the first time that the child inhales air from the environment outside the mother's body. It marks the end of the life that depended on the uterus, and provides the impetus to function independently, becoming the interface between the ever-changing external environment and the constantly maintained internal environment of the body. The effects of the breath infiltrate every single cell of the body, but are most essential for the brain, which uses up a great proportion of the oxygen.

The movements of breathing and the motion of primary respiration are influenced by each other. A good breath comes from the diaphragm and spreads throughout the body, something best seen in animals and newborn babies. Somehow, as we grow older we forget what it was like to breathe properly and end up usually breathing from the upper chest. Breathing in is an active, conscious process involving muscular activity, while breathing out is the elastic recoil of the lungs and the chest wall with relaxation of its muscles. Breathing movements are influenced by posture – having a good stretch allows the lungs to expand, with an automatic urge to breathe in. The opposite occurs when we are slumped so that the lungs feel small and it becomes difficult to breathe in.

Although breathing is an automatic act, we can control the messages to the respiratory muscles to alter the rate and depth of the breath. The yogis have an ancient tradition of controlling the flow of the 'prana' or life force and slowing down the ageing process. From this we can surmise that with practice the breath may be used as a regenerative force and a means of controlling other processes such as blood pressure and heart beat. Emotions do affect our breathing, but often in a less than useful way. When there is anger or anxiety over a long period of time, the compensating physiological processes tend to maintain these effects in the body. Breathing becomes shallow, fast and irregular and this is reflected in the mind starting to feel unsteady. Chest breathing, as opposed to breathing from the abdomen, is actually a part of the stress response, and brings about tension and anxiety, which in time can lead to high blood pressure and other problems. Since the lower lobes of the lungs are abundantly supplied with blood, chest breathing means they are not ventilated properly and there is poor gas exchange between the air in the lungs and the blood. With time this can affect the levels of oxygen taken into the body. But if we are happy, feeling secure, laughing, it is likely that the breath is deeper.

Tips

• Make a habit of spending time on breathing consciously and just being still for some minutes. Try to keep it at a regular time and at a still place each day. Breath awareness is a reliable method for preparing for meditation and helps the mind to become focused. In time, it helps to bring a vast part of the unconscious mind, including memory, under conscious control. Through constant awareness of the breath the mind can be trained to remain in the present rather than flitting between moments gone and those to come. By being aware of the now we allow ourselves to experience an essential part of eternity.

- It is a good idea to spend a few minutes each day concentrating on an even flow of breathing in and out. Sit with a straight back in a chair and begin by breathing from the abdomen and lower lungs only. Place one hand on the upper abdomen and the other on the upper chest. As you breathe in, the lower hand should rise up. With deeper and increasing breath, gradually the upper hand will rise up.
- Another way is to spread your hands on either side of the lower part of the rib cage so that the lower sides are filled up. Gradually bring this breath up to the upper lobes of the lungs, but without moving the shoulders.
- Self-help measures of meditation, biofeedback, visualization and yoga help the body to become rebalanced.
- Try to spend some time out of doors, in touch with the natural world. You may or may not wish to incorporate this with breathing practice.
- Remember the saying 'laughter is the best medicine'. A good hearty laugh mobilizes everything, including mood-enhancing endorphins. Apparently it takes 42 muscles to frown and only 28 to smile!

In times of acute stress or when you are feeling overwhelmed by deadlines, tell yourself that this period will eventually be over. Either your body will give in or you will; realize that somewhere changes need to be made! But when you cannot see when that change is going to happen:

- Try to ensure that you are among people who love and support you. This should include people who can freely hug you, and children are great at this.
- As mentioned above, never let the fridge go empty – this will help you look after yourself when times are hard.
- Try to work with focus, for hourly or two-hourly slots, with natural breaks for nibbles or just to practise breathing consciously.
- Unwind at the end of the day with a walk or some physical activity: this will help to release the happy endorphins. Once the stressful period is over you can then enrol in the stress-control, yoga or meditation class. In time these techniques will come naturally and become habitual, so that when the next stressful period occurs (and it will) the body has a greater buffer zone to counter it.

An exercise for balancing the cranium, spine and sacrum

There are over 30 muscles attached to the base of the skull and connected to the spine. In addition, there are fascial tissues that go right down to the feet and all have a bearing on the motions of primary respiration. This exercise is to help to release the tension in these soft tissues and to elongate the neck, spine and pelvis, which have become compressed from the effects of being upright. It is especially useful if you feel run down and have low energy levels.

Lie on your back, with the knees bent up and hands at either side resting on the floor or on the chest. The head lies on the edge of a pile of books about 10 centimetres (4 inches) high. The contact point is at the back of the head where there is a bumpy area. If this is too sore, put a towel over the books to soften the edge. Stay still for about twenty minutes each day. You can concentrate on the breath or listen to music in this time, but nothing else.

Spinal twists

Most of our actions are habitual so we tend to use the same set of muscles. We generally perform most of our functions by bending forwards and even fitness routines such as running only involve anterior/posterior actions. This exercise gives the body a chance to look at things from a different perspective, by introducing a twisting motion into the spine and its attached soft tissues.

Lie on the floor with the knees bent up. Then allow them to fall to one side, while turning the head and both arms to the opposite side. Hold for as long as is comfortable, until you feel the tissues stretching. Come back to the starting posture and then repeat the exercise by letting the bent knees fall to the other side and moving the head and arms to the opposite side. After a while, crossing one leg over the other can make this exercise a bit harder. For example, cross the right leg over the left and allow the legs to fall to the right (to the side of the leg on top). This will exaggerate the hip, pelvic and spinal stretch.

Appendix 1

THE VERTEBRAL COLUMN

Every area of the body is controlled by nerves. The normal function of these nerves can be disturbed by misalignments of the vertebrae affecting the specific areas, as shown below:

	AREA	EFFECTS
C1	Blood supply to the head, the pituitary gland, the scalp, bones of the face, the brain itself, inner and middle ear, the sympathetic nervous system	Headaches, migraine headaches, nervousness, insomnia, high blood pressure, amnesia, chronic tiredness, dizziness, vertigo, St Vitus dance
C2	Eyes, optic nerve, auditory nerve, sinuses, mastoid bones, tongue, forehead	Sinus trouble, allergies, crossed eyes, erysipelas, eye troubles, earache, certain cases of blindness
C3	Cheeks, outer ear, face bones, teeth, trifacial nerve	Neuralgia, neuritis, acne or pimples
C4	Nose, lips, mouth, eustachian tube	Hay fever, catarrh, hearing problems
C5	Vocal cords, neck glands, pharynx	Laryngitis, hoarseness, throat conditions, sore throat
C6	Neck muscles, shoulders, tonsils	Stiff neck, pain in upper arm, tonsillitis, whooping cough, croup
C7	Thyroid gland, bursae in the shoulders, the elbows	Bursitis, colds, thyroid conditions
T1	Arms from the elbows down, including the hands, wrists and fingers, also the oesophagus and trachea	Asthma, coughs, difficult breathing, shortness of breath, pain in lower arms and hands
T2	Heart including its valves and covering, also coronary arteries	Functional heart conditions and certain pains
T3	Lungs, bronchial tubes, pleura, chest, breast, nipples	Bronchitis, pleurisy, pneumonia, congestion, influenza
T4	Gall bladder and common duct	Gall bladder conditions, jaundice, shingles

Vertebra	Body parts	Conditions
T5	Liver, solar plexus, blood	Liver conditions, fevers, low blood pressure, anaemia, poor circulation, arthritis
T6	Stomach	Stomach troubles including nervous stomach, poor digestion, heart burn, dyspepsia
T7	Pancreas, islands of Lengerhans, duodenum	Diabetes, ulcers, gastritis
T8	Spleen, diaphragm	Hiccups, lowered resistance
T9	Adrenals or supra-renals	Allergies, hives
T10	Kidneys	Kidney troubles, hardening of the arteries, chronic tiredness, nephritis, pyelitis
T11	Kidneys, uretera	Skin conditions such as acne, pimples, eczema, boils
T12	Small intestine, Fallopian tubes, lymph circulation	Rheumatism, wind pains
L1	Large intestine, inguinal rings	Constipation, colitis, dysentery, diarrhoea, hernias
L2	Appendix, abdomen, upper leg, caecum	Appendicitis, cramps, difficulty in breathing, varicose veins
L3	Sex organs, ovaries or testicles, uterus, bladder, knee	Bladder troubles, menstrual problems, miscarriages, bedwetting, impotence, change of life symptoms
L4	Prostate gland, muscles of the lower back, sciatic nerve	Sciatica, lumbago, difficult, painful or too frequent urination, backaches
L5	Lower legs, ankles, feet, toes, arches	Poor circulation in the legs, swollen ankles, cold feet, weakness in the legs, leg cramps
sacrum	Hip bones, buttocks	Sacroiliac conditions, spinal curvatures
coccyx	Rectum, anus	Haemorrhoids (piles), pruritus (itching), discomfort at end of spine on sitting

The evolving concept of osteopathy in the cranial field

The practice of using hands to assist the natural healing processes of the body is not new: the laying on of hands, massage with or without the use of oils and manipulation of the joints were well known as scientific and esoteric practices to the ancient traditions throughout the world. The application of touch as a means of healing the other senses, including the mind, are well documented in the ancient Indian Ayurvedic texts of Sutrasthana Caraka-Samhita, while Hippocrates describes spinal manipulation in *Corpus Hippocrateum*. From the Middle Ages to the late nineteenth century, in Europe and later in America, a combination of massage with manipulation became the domain of the 'bone-setter'.

Osteopathy introduced to the Western world in 1874 by Dr Andrew Taylor Still was a culmination of different influences. In the mid-1700s, John Wesley and Methodism advocated nature cures, simple medicines and the virtues of wholesome food, exercise and cleanliness. George Coombe, in his 'Essay on The Constitution of Man, Considered in relation to External Objects' (1828), which looked at the structure of the human being and his ability to move, wrote: 'The Creator has bestowed on him bones, muscles and nerves, constructed on the most perfect principles, which enable him to preserve, and adapt his movements to gravity.' Then in the 1850s phrenologists demonstrated a science of natural law illustrating human and animal progression through skulls and plaster casts of brains. They taught that the human body was a part of the universe and that the health and mind would improve by following the governing laws of the universe. These laws related to the perfection and completeness of the organized being, the need for a supply of food, light, air and other physical requirements for the body's support, and for exercise as a prerequisite for health.

By the time Still was thinking about these new ideas in healing, the phrenology movement was gradually overtaken by an Austrian idea, mesmerism, named after Franz Anton Mesmer who in 1772 had also originally introduced the idea of the healing properties of magnets. Later, from the late 1830s, magnetic healers combined their practices with those of phrenology, hypnosis and eventually with electricity. But an American eclectic, Joseph Rodes Buchanan, went further in combining phrenology with Franz Joseph Gall's theory (1819) of special areas in the brain relating to functions in the physical organs (neurology): he wrote, 'every organ of the body is directed by a separate region of the brain by means of "nervaura" . . . Moreover, every passion or emotion and every function performed in the body has a legitimate origin in some part of the nervous system.' He used manipulation to conduct the nervous or cerebral fluid radiating from the brain to the organs of the body.

During the latter half of the nineteenth century, the theory of evolution and Charles Darwin's *The Origin of Species* dominated scientific thought. However, it was the English philosopher Herbert Spencer who in his *First Principles* (1862) made the concept of natural selection palatable to Americans. Spencer had a huge impact on Still. Spencer saw evolution as a natural law applied on every scale, where all species are progressing towards perfection; he emphasized the inter-relation of cause and effect, structure and function, the specialization of functions, and the mutual dependence of the parts as well as the interconnectedness of the universe. He used simple analogies such as the evolution of the bowstring to a harp or the egg to the chicken to describe the constant state of tension in which the universe was evolving from the simple to the complex.

Still's work reflects the mechanistic model of much nineteenth-century science: the fundamental principles of osteopathy are that structure and function are inter-related. Yet Still, like Spencer, was convinced of evolutionary progress towards perfection – and for him, the idea of perfection was expressive of God. His ideas continued to develop until in 1874 he wrote:

> I was shot . . . not in the heart, but in the dome of reason. The dome was then in a very poor condition to be penetrated by an arrow charged with the principles of philosophy . . . I saw by the force of reason that the word 'God' signified perfection in all things and in all places. I began at that date to carefully examine with the microscope of mind to prove an assertion that is often made . . . that the perfection of Deity can be proven by his Works.

In 1898, William Garner Sutherland came to study osteopathy as taught by Dr Still and this resulted in a lifetime's work that now forms the basis of osteopathy in the cranial field. Still had always emphasized that the articulations of the bones were designed for motion. While examining the different bones of the skull Sutherland realized they too were designed for motion and indeed could be separated from each other. He observed that there were different types of surfaces for articulation amongst the different bones of the skull. The bevel and angles even changed from one side of the bone to provide 'mechanical facility for gliding motion', 'rock-shaft bearing', or 'a combined rock-shaft pivot bearing providing rotation and undulation' of the different bones.

The thinking of that time was that the bones of the adult skull had become fused – so, troubled, Sutherland set out to disprove his own findings. He made up various straps and contraptions to ensure that any potential movement between the cranial and facial bones would be inhibited. He soon made himself quite ill suffering with headaches, disorientation and nausea (among other symptoms). He came to realize that there had to be motion between the bones of the skull and that this motion played an important role in the functioning of the total body physiology. (This period of his work was, broadly, between 1898 and 1929.) The idea of cranial movement was not unknown in the Eastern traditions: Indian midwives, for example, were well versed in crude cranial manipulation and resetting of the bones after delivery.

Sutherland found that the brain also had its own intrinsic motion, his conclusions (1937) having borne out the experiments of an eighteenth-century scientist, Emanuel Swedenborg. In addition, Sutherland believed the cerebrospinal fluid of the brain and spinal cord had a fluctuating movement which was quite independent of its circulatory movements.

Sutherland went on to discover that the motion of the bones was intrinsic since muscles did not move them. He was initially searching for the physical manifestations of bony motion and reasoned, in line with the mechanical osteopathic model of the time, that because of the continuity of the cranial and spinal membranes, the inherent motions of the bones occurred through tension created in them. The correction techniques therefore employed the use of membranous tension to create levers on the bony strains. The following is a description by Sutherland of Still's approach to technique, which also indicates how Sutherland was developing and extending his thinking about the cranial mechanism:

> In technique we endeavour to follow Dr Still's methods. That is, getting the point of release with no jerking and then allowing the natural agencies to return the bones to their normal relations and positions. What are the natural agencies? The ligaments, not the muscles, are the natural agencies for this purpose of correcting relations and positions of the joints. Dr Still's application of the technique is the gentle exaggeration of the lesion that allows the natural agencies to draw the bones into place . . . There is reason for applying that technique in the cranial mechanism. The difference between spinal technique is like the difference between the automobile mechanic and a watch maker. We do not force anything into place in the reduction of the lesion. We have something more potent than our own forces working always in the patient towards the direction of the normal.

The 'normal agencies' in the cranium were the brain, which was the motor of respiration, the cerebrospinal fluid and the tension in the membranes. The inborn ability of the brain to move spontaneously and the inherent fluctuation of its fluid seemed to coincide with changes in the shape of the cranium. Sutherland thought of these motions as being expressed and felt as alternating contractile and expansile movements, similar to those of the chest when breathing in and out. Possibly because of the cranial bones' capacity for articular motion, these changes in shape could be accommodated. The cranial and spinal membranes provided a tension mechanism, while the cerebrospinal fluid provided a fluid drive and a hydraulic system. Consequently, motions in the sacrum could be felt as well as those in the cranium. Sutherland viewed the combination of these factors as a 'primary respiratory mechanism', whose manifested rhythmic alternating motions were independent of breathing from the chest and diaphragm.

The term 'primary respiration' gave an indication that the physiological centres that control and regulate the life processes, including breathing, were to be found in the brain stem and were therefore of primary importance. Dr Harold I. Magoun has stated that 'physiological respiration is metabolism, the giving off of waste material and the formation of new by the cellular protoplasm. Metabolism is further defined as a tissue change, the sum of the chemical changes whereby the function of nutrition is effected. It consists of anabolism and catabolism.' What Sutherland meant by the primary respiratory mechanism was a 'metabolic and regulatory complex'; this is the breathing of each individual cell or internal respiration, which occurs through the exchange of respiratory gases between the tissue cells and their internal environment.

But what was the origin of these motions? Still, while philosophizing how the channelling of the Universal Intelligence might reach the fundamentals of human physiology, felt that 'the cerebrospinal fluid is the highest known element in the human body, and unless the brain furnishes this fluid in abundance, a disabled condition of the body will remain . . . this great river of life must be tapped and the withering field irrigated at once, or the harvest of health be forever lost.'

And so, after decades of study into cranial motion within the body, Sutherland concurred with Still's view that the cerebrospinal fluid receives the Universal Intelligence. He endowed it with the name 'Breath of Life', which he took to be the animating essence of primary respiration. In other words, the alternating rhythmic contractile and expansile motions of the cranial articular structures were the primary physiological effects of the Breath of Life or the universal intention in action. By 1943, he was describing the Breath of Life as the 'initiative spark' and organizer for the central nervous system and its fluid. It was responsible for the creation of form and function of the human body, which became the fundamental principle in the cranial concept: 'the Breath of Life, not the breath of air, was breathed into the nasals of this form of clay and man became a living soul to walk about on earth and utilize one of its living elements . . . the breath of air.' (This reference was to Genesis 2:7, King James's Version: 'and breathed into his nostrils the breath of life, and man became a living soul.')

Sutherland's explorations of bony motion (1944–8) led him to discover more subtle, fluid motions. The Breath of Life had Universal Intelligence and the effects were not just limited to the physical form but encompassed everything. It generated a supreme potency and could be felt by the hands as 'an invisible "fluid" within the cerebrospinal fluid'. Magoun describes it as 'the mechanical power inherent within the cerebrospinal fluid as a body of liquid, which is not compressible . . . ' and because of this 'the hydrodynamic relationship with the rest of the body automatically extends this inherent power throughout the organism.'

Sutherland's experiments began by trying to disprove his own ideas, and moved on to a lifetime's work in exploring the natural state of the fluid motion within the body. In so doing, he moved from the mechanistic model to a more dynamic model of viewing the workings of the body. He saw fluids in all the systems: 'What are bones but fluid, a different form of fluid? What is that little hailstone that comes down from heaven but fluid? What is this . . . world that we walk on, but fluid?' 'Take a can of water and give it a shake and set it down. Place your hand on the can and you will feel the water within it fluctuate. You can feel such a movement in the cranium.' The potency within fluids was to be found somewhere in the mid-point of the alternating motions of primary respiration. Sutherland likened it to the invisible X-ray, where the equipment can be seen, but not the ray, which makes the picture by exposing the film, or like sheet lightning that lights up the cloud, but does not touch it. This idea of potency within the fluids is an important tool in some of the technical procedures used today by osteopaths in the cranial field.

Sutherland was more than just working with the anatomical and physiological considerations of the cerebrospinal fluid, and its nature in health, trauma and disease. Towards the time of his death in 1954, he was feeling within the cerebrospinal fluid an invisible and yet palpable 'liquid light' with the capacity of transmutation. So, the capacity of the Breath of Life (animating essence of primary respiration) in physiological terms means that it creates motion through the bioelectric, biomolecular and biomechanical components of the body. With transmutation, then, occurred a change within all of these fields. The ability of the body to transmute is a naturally occurring phenomenon that goes on throughout life. The synthesis of adenosine triphosphate (ATP) as an energy currency from eating a grape, the formation of urine, the healing of a wound, or a recall of a memory from a familiar smell are all basic examples of daily transmutation. In using potency within the fluids as a tool this process was phenomenally enhanced. Within the cerebrosopinal fluid, it generates a cellular interchange of the hormones, neurones, lymphatics and other cellular and fluid systems of the body.

Sutherland's explorations were many and original, but they were based on the work of Still, which itself was far ahead of their time. Throughout his life, Sutherland's ideas of the nature of primary respiration were constantly evolving and becoming refined. Many have followed his work and made some remarkable contributions to the field. Rollin Becker was a student of Sutherland. Amongst other things, his notions of primary respiration explored the impact of the immediate environment or 'biosphere'. He referred to the Breath of Life as the 'Long Tide' that was more easily felt and appreciated outside of the body. The primary influence on growth and development and subsequent health is known to be the environment. Becker was looking at the interchange of motions felt not only within the body, but also with the environment. He saw how the impact of physical forces of trauma, for example, modified the body physiology by distorting the cellular fluids and hence their membranous walls. The result was not only an altered capacity of movement of the body, but also of altered motion within the tissues of the body and unless the vectors of these forces were addressed, resolution and hence healing was only partial.

The ever-evolving model of Sutherland's work continued to be studied by many, including a group of osteopaths in New England. Using their perceptual skills to focus on the natural laws and the kinetics of motion these practitioners came to realize that the pattern of motions felt by so many osteopaths were similar to the direction and shape of motions in which embryonic growth occurs. The alternate rhythmic motions, which were clinically perceptible, were the inherent basic rhythm of the developing organism. What is responsible for the formation of the early weeks of embryonic life, until three to four weeks, is largely unknown, but by the eighth week embryonic formation is completed. Dr James Jealous reviewed the work of Sutherland and fluid motion in relation to the work of a German embryologist, Blechschmidt. Blechschmidt's remarkable book entitled *The Beginning of Human Life* refuted the established phylogenetic considerations of human embryology. The work was based on the morphological investigations of human embryos (between 1942 and 1972) and had two striking features:

1 In order to show the early differentiation, the author had taken an extraordinary series of freeze-dried embryos two to three days apart in age. He then sliced through them and drew them as a series of succeeding stages of development. He also made cardboard/polyester models and out of them revealed an expression of a functional motion. This showed that the embryo developed as a single unit rather than as a number of isolated parts and that developmental movements occurring in one region were related to those occurring simultaneously in neighbouring regions.

2 The development of the organs, such as the heart or stomach, was shown by the changes of shape, structure and position as movements occurring in metabolic fields. The position, shape and structure were kinetically related throughout development. Blechschmidt's published work (1961, 1977) described embryology as a series of three-dimensional organizations of interchanging metabolic fields in motion, which refuted the traditional views of embryology.

Working in the 1960s, the New England group of osteopaths saw Blechschmidt's work, and in his depictions of embryonic development began to recognize that the patterns of motion they felt through their hands were those of the developing embryo. They were feeling the motion of the embryological forces that developed the human being. The organizing force of the 'original design and function' was present in the fluids of the embryo and did not come from the genetic influences. It is as if the embryo itself contained the idea of the form of the body and brought it into being. For example, prior to the development of an arm (at about 28 days of gestation) there is a fluid idea, then a field or shape, into which the arm will grow, first in cartilage and then in bone. The developmental pattern of the embryo's limb bud behaves in the adult as if mimicking the pregenetic or embryological developmental pattern. Whilst Blechschmidt was describing the different ways in which fluids interact with each other inside the body, Sutherland perceived these same forces in the fluids and yet the two had never read each other's work. Jealous put these two ideas together and out of this connection grew 'biodynamics of osteopathy in the cranial field', which acknowledges the underlying organizing force, Jealous having used the term the 'Original matrix' to describe this manifestation.

Philosophically, the notion of an organizing life force present in all living tissues is very old. Blechschmidt had shown the presence of formative forces – the generative forces that form the embryo. During development these forces created form and function and were dynamic – therefore, as Jealous puts it, 'everything, including blood sugar, has spatial dynamics'. These formative forces always stay present and are thought to be responsible for sustaining the normal functions such as those of the heart and lungs and for the repair of the body. So, for example, the organizing life force maintains the capacity of the central nervous system to function normally in someone who has a concussion, or for repairing a broken leg. When palpating the original developmental forces with the hands, the osteopath can observe their therapeutic effects – for example, in making therapeutic use of forces that are outside the central nervous system in conditions of head injury, concussion and even cerebral palsy. The same embryological forces were hypothesized as healing and sustaining in themselves, and it was thought that health would be encouraged by supporting those forces. According to Jealous:

> The breath of life forms life, perfectly, then the form is modified by generic and cultural forces. We can perceive the breath of life come into the body, come to the midline, and from the midline, generate different forms of rhythms in the bioelectric field, fluids and tissues. Essentially what is happening is genesis. It never stops. Moment to moment we are building new form and function. One senses this directly.

And:

> Health can be defined as the emergence of Originality. The Originality expresses a complete balance of both structure and function as intentionalized in the creation of the human being. This Health . . . is at the core of our being and cannot be increased or decreased . . . this

Original matrix within the human body interfaces with every physiological, structural and psychological stress that one contacts. This interface begins early as our encounter with our genetics and ends at death with a shift in our perceptual field. It is the existence of this background that allows osteopathic physicians to palpate a nonverbal history on their patients.

Osteopathy in the cranial field as envisaged by Sutherland is an ever-evolving process. As new information becomes available about physiology and the natural laws, they add credence to the incredible insight of the forefathers of osteopathy. With additional knowledge the model may change again, as it has previously done, from a biomechanical to a biodynamic model. For example, there has been much research into the nature of water and the ability to hold memory. According to the studies of the French scientist Benveniste during the 1980s, water is essential to the transmission of energy and information through molecular signals. The body and all living things contain water; in a process called 'super-radiance', water as the natural medium of all cells acts as a conductor of a molecule's signature frequency in all biological processes. The organization of the water molecules is such that they form a pattern upon which can be imprinted wave information and this may be one reason why the body can continue to exhibit its embryonic motion patterns, as palpated by osteopaths using the biodynamic model.

In addition, the universe is also revealing its secrets and numerous scientists like Americans Timothy Boyer and Hal Puthoff using quantum calculations have shown that we, and our universe, live and breathe in a sea of motion. There is a background field, known as a matrix or medium and referred to as the 'zero point field', which is a repository of all fields, all ground energy states and all virtual particles. This field is an ocean of vibrations or waves that appears to connect everything in the universe and seems to hold all of its information in the form of waves. It also seems to contain large quantum energy present in dead space or the space between things. This is because, with every exchange between virtual particles there is a radiation of energy, which when added together becomes a vast inexhaustible energy source. A number of scientists have discovered that all living beings emit a weak radiation as a result of biological processes, so they are therefore essentially packets of quantum energy constantly exchanging information with the inexhaustible energy sea. This implies an information exchange on a quantum level about all aspects of life, from cellular communication to thinking and feeling, so that human perception becomes an interaction between the subatomic particles of the brain and the quantum energy sea. This gives a basis on which we resonate with our world – and one of the tenets of osteopathy is the relationship of the physical body with the environment. The coherence created by the zero point field waves may reveal the interconnectedness of all of us to our universe.

While these theories are academic, they also take us back to Herbert Spencer, who saw evolution as a progression towards perfection and who wrote of the interconnectedness of everything within the universe. He defined evolution as:

> An integration of matter and concomitant dissipation of motion; during which the matter passes from a relatively indefinite, incoherent homogeneity to a relative, definite, coherent heterogeneity, and during which the retained motion undergoes a parallel transformation.

In using primary respiration as a therapeutic tool, the osteopath can feel this transformation and homogeneity of the tissues as they normalize their function. Although we may develop theories about healing using natural forces, the nature of primary respiration and the Breath of Life is still a mystery, which reveals glimpses of its intension and power to the osteopath through her own stillness. Her evolution is through her individual experience based on the skills of perception and touch. And as the osteopath herself evolves, more is revealed to her of the Breath of Life that created form and of the Intelligence behind primary respiration.

What makes cranial osteopathy different from other therapies using the cranial approach?

A question I am often asked is 'What is the difference between cranial osteopathy and cranio-sacral therapy?' Cranio-sacral therapy was a term introduced by Dr John Upledger, an osteopath who had the opportunity to view the motion of the cranial membranes whilst assisting in a routine spinal surgery in 1970, described in his book Your Inner Physician and You. Fascinated by the motion that Sutherland had originally described, Upledger researched it extensively in order to prove its existence scientifically. He saw the clinical benefit of cranial osteopathy and felt that it should be made accessible to everyone and not remain the sole domain of osteopaths. Thus in order to teach a wider group of students he put together a system that took some procedures used in cranial osteopathy, added to them and has since popularized this as a therapy. Indeed, many other healthcare practitioners using hands-on work have absorbed some of the technical procedures of osteopathy in the cranial field. Unless the patient has some background knowledge of these fields, he is often hard put to be able to differentiate between, for example, chiropractic craniopathy, sacro-occipital techniques, energetic healing and other biodynamic approaches. Each approach has its own rationale, and those interested in finding out more about them may want to do some research through the internet. A great deal of material about cranio-sacral therapy is availalable through the Upledger Institute, based in the USA (www.upledger.com).

I am also often asked about what sort of training osteopaths undergo. Osteopaths have a rigorous training programme, which is often one of the reasons why patients are confident in seeking osteopathy out or in being referred for treatment. Throughout Britain, Europe and Australia, an osteopath practising in the cranial field will have undergone extensive training over a four to five year period leading to degree status, with the opportunity for research. She will have studied in depth (among other subjects) applied anatomy, physiology and pathology as well as osteopathic philosophy and principles. The situation is somewhat different in America where the training leads to a medical doctorate. So the American osteopath will bring with her a knowledge of surgery, drugs, psychology and other sciences as a result of internship and residency programmes, in addition to the cranial work. To specialize further in the cranial procedures, the osteopath will have undergone post-graduate education under the umbrella organization of the Sutherland Cranial Teaching Foundation. If she then wants to specialize in the osteopathic care of children, the Osteopathic Centre for Children in London offers a two-year programme leading to a diploma in paediatric osteopathy.

An osteopath is legally licensed and regulated, certainly in Britain, Australia and America. The government bodies ensure the quality and training of the osteopath as well as the safety and practice of osteopathy, and the practitioner is liable for her actions.

Dr Sutherland was adamant that osteopathy in the cranial field was built upon the foundation of osteopathic understanding and knowledge. An osteopath who practises in the cranial field brings the ability to make an informed diagnosis and base her treatment using primary respiration upon the background of her established training and professional credentials.

Where to find out about osteopathy

UNITED KINGDOM

The General Osteopathic Council
Osteopathy House
176 Tower Bridge Road
London SE1 3LU
Tel: 020 7357 6655 (ext. 242)
www.osteopathy.org.uk

The Sutherland Cranial College
Spring Vale
Mill Hill
Brockweir
Gloucester
NP6 7NW
Tel: 01291 689908
email:
suthcranialcoll@compuserve.com

The Sutherland Society
Helen Allison
Still Point Clinic
13a Hyde Road
Denton
Manchester
Tel: 0161 336 6666
www.cranial.org.uk

Osteopathic Centre for Children
109 Harley Street
London
W1G 6AN
Tel: 020 7486 6160

UNITED STATES OF AMERICA

American Academy of Osteopathy
3500 DePauw Boulevard
Suite 1080
Indianapolis
IN 46268-1136

American Osteopathic Association
142 East Ontario Street
Chicago
IL 60611
Tel: 312 280 5580
Fax: 312 280 3860
email:info@aoa.net.org
www.am-osteo-assn.org

The Cranial Academy
8202 Clearvista Parkway
Suite 9-D
Indianapolis
IN 46256
Tel: 317 594 0411
Fax: 317 594 9299

Sutherland Cranial Teaching
   Foundation, Inc.,
4116 Hartwood Drive,
Fort Worth, Texas 76109
Tel: 817 926 7705

Osteopathic Centre for Children
630 Gentre
La Jolla
Ca 92037 5422

AUSTRALIA

Australian Osteopathic
  Association
AOA Federal Office
PO Box 242
Thornleigh
NSW 2120
Tel: 61 2 9440 2511
Fax: 61 2 9440 9962
http:/www.osteopathic.com.au

NEW ZEALAND

New Zealand Register of
  Osteopaths
PO Box 14697
Wellington
Tel: 64 4 970 3454
Fax: 64 4 970 3454

AUSTRIA

Austrian delegation of the
  European Register of Osteopaths
Jagdschlongasse 40/2/1
1130 Wien
Tel: 43 1 804 2929
Fax: 43 1 333 8340

FRANCE

Register des Ostéopathes
  de France
22 rue Fondande
33000 Bordeaux
Tel: 0033 556 6009009
Fax: 0033 556 6009010
www.osteopathie.org

GERMANY

The Sutherland Society
Eva Moeckel
Heilpraktikerin Osteopathin
Goethehealle 6
Tel: 0049 40 4905864

Reading list

REFERENCES FOR PRACTITIONERS

Armitage, Peter, D.O. 'Tensegrity' (unpublished paper)
Becker, Rollin E., D.O. 'Life in Motion', *The Osteopathic Vision of Rollin E. Becker, D.O.*, Rudra Press, Portland, 1997
— 'Stillness of Life' *The Osteopathic Philosophy of Rollin E. Becker, D.O.*, Stillness Press, USA, 2000
Blechschmidt, E., M.D. & R.F. Gasser, Ph.D. *Biokinetics and Biodynamics of Human Differentiation: Principles and Applications*, Charles C. Thomas, Springfield, Illinois, 1978
Frymann, Viola M., D.O. *The Collected Papers of Viola M. Frymann, D.O.: Legacy of Osteopathy to Children*, American Academy of Osteopathy, Indianapolis, 1998
Handoll, Nicholas, D.O. *Anatomy of Potency*, Osteopathic Supplies Limited, Hereford, 2000
Magoun, Harold Ives, A.B., D.O., M.Sc. *Osteopathy in the Cranial Field*, 1st edition 1951, Sutherland Cranial Teaching Foundation, Kirksville, Missouri, 1997
Pottenger, Francis Marion, A.M., M.D., LL.D., F.A.C.P. *Symptoms of Visceral Disease*, 6th edition, C.V. Mosby Company, St Louis, 1949
Still, Andrew Taylor *Autobiography of A. T. Still*, American Academy of Osteopathy, Kirksville, Missouri, 1908, 3rd reprint 1994
— *The Philosophy and Mechanical Principles of Osteopathy*, Osteopathic Enterprise, Kirksville, Missouri, 1986
Sutherland, William Garner, D.O. *Contributions of Thought*, 2nd edition, Rudra Press, Portland, 1998
Swedenborg, Emanuel *The Cerebrum and its Parts*, Vol. 1 of *The Brain Considered Anatomically, Physiologically*, Swedenborg Scientific Association, 1938
Trowbridge, Carol *Andrew Taylor Still 1828–1917*, Thomas Jefferson University Press, Kirksville, Missouri, 1991

FOR A LESS HEAVY READ

Fulford, Robert C., D.O. & Gene Stone *Dr Fulford's Touch of Life*, Pocket Books, New York, 1996
Hayden, Elizabeth C., D.O. *Osteopathy for Children*, 3rd edition, Elizabeth C. Hayden, UK, 2000
Jealous, James S. 'Healing in the Natural World' in *Alternative Therapies in Medicine*, Innovisions Communications Vol. 1, Encinitas, California, January 1977

Levinson, Daniel *The Seasons of a Man's Life*, Knopf, New York, 1978

McTaggart, Lynne *The Field: the Quest for the Secret Force of the Universe*, HarperCollins, London, 2001

Moody Harry R. & Davis Carrol *The Five Stages of the Soul*, Rider, London, 1999

Pert, Candace B., Ph.D. *Molecules of Emotion: Why You Feel the Way You Feel*, Pocket Books, New York, 1999

Saplosky, Robert M. *Why Zebras Don't Get Ulcers: An Updated Guide to Stress, Stress-Related Diseases, and Coping*, Freeman, New York, 1998

Verny, Thomas, M.D. & John Kelly *The Secret Life of the Unborn Child: How You Can Prepare Your Unborn Baby for a Happy, Healthy Life*, Time Warner, New York, 1988

SELF-HELP BOOKS

Clark, Jane *Bodyfoods Cookbook*, Cassell, London, 2001

Gelb, Harold, D.M.D. & Paula M. Siegel *Killing Pain Without Prescription: A New and Simple Way to Free Yourself from Headache, Backache and Other Sources of Chronic Pain*, Thorsons, London, 1984

Khalsa, Gurmukh Kaur *The Eight Human Talents: The Yoga Way to Restore Balance and Serenity Within*, Thorsons, London, 2000

Page, Christine & Keith Hagenbach *Mind, Body, Spirit Workbook: A Handbook of Health*, The C.W. Daniel Company Ltd, Saffron Walden, 1999

Pitchford, Paul *Healing With Whole Foods: Oriental Traditions and Modern Nutrition*, North Atlantic Books, Berkeley, California,1993

Rama, Swami, Rudolph Ballentine, M.D. & Alan Hymes, M.D. *Science of Breath: A Practical Guide*, Himalayan Institute, Honesdale, Pennsylvania, 1988

Wheater, Caroline *Juicing for Health*, Thorsons, London, 1993

Index